EVOLVING TRENDS IN UROLOGY

Edited by **Sashi S. Kommu**

Evolving Trends in Urology
Edited by Sashi S. Kommu

Published by InTech
Janeza Trdine 9, 51000 Rijeka, Croatia

Publishing Process Manager Oliver Kurelic

Technical Editor Teodora Smiljanic

Cover Designer InTech Design Team

Additional hard copies can be obtained from orders@intechopen.com

Evolving Trends in Urology, Edited by Sashi S. Kommu
p. cm.
ISBN 978-953-51-0811-5

For EU product safety concerns:
IN TECH d.o.o., Prolaz Marije Krucifikse Kozulić 3, 51000 Rijeka, Croatia, info@intechopen.com or visit our website at intechopen.com.

Meet the editor

Dr Sashi Sekhar Kommu was recently appointed as the youngest member of the Advisory Consultant Board for SCIYO, one of the largest and fastest-growing open access scientific publishers in the world. He is a member of all four colleges of The Royal College of Surgeons in the United Kingdom. He completed his Basic Surgical Training in the North West in England and is currently training as a Specialist Registrar/ Urology Resident in the London Deanery in the United Kingdom. At the age of 8 he developed his first robot, 'Microman' which was programmed to water his father's garden. Nine years later he was admitted to Medical School where he fulfilled his life long passion to follow in his father's footsteps (Dr Rajeswara Rao Kommu) as a doctor. His academic interests are both clinical and basic sciences. His key clinical interests are in the minimally invasive treatment of urological cancers, surgical robotics and intelligent probes. He has done formal research at The Royal Marsden NHS Foundation Trust and The Institute of Cancer Research with The Translational Cancer Genetics Team where he refined his scientific methodology in advanced labarotory work with an emphasis on cancer genetics and proteomics. He has also gained vast exposure in Nanotechnology. He has over 90 peer-reviewed publications in respected scientific and medical journals including The Lancet. He also has over 280 Scientific Presentations, several book chapters and books. Dr Kommu has over 25 academic awards including The Olympus Award at The 25th World Congress of Endourology in Cleveland U.S.A. 2006. He has nine patents pending including, a cost effective Telerounding Kit for Remote Teleconsultations, which was presented at The House of Commons (Hosted by The British Parliament) in 2006. His ability to blend medical science with engineering and technology has earned him two NASA collaborative scientific commendations. Dr Kommu is reviewer for 15 Surgical/Urological and 3 Basic Sciences Journals. Among several novel concepts described by Dr Kommu, include 'suppressor screening in urological cancer screening' and 'the supplementary biomarker approach' for detecting cancers.

Contents

Preface IX

Chapter 1 **Telementoring and Telerobotics in Urological Surgery 1**
Yasmin Abu-Ghanem, Sarah Wheatstone and Benjamin Challacombe

Chapter 2 **Febrile Urinary Tract Infections in Children Less Than 2 Years of Age 15**
Pavel Geier and Janusz Feber

Chapter 3 **Evolving Role of Simulators and Training in Robotic Urological Surgery 21**
Sashi S. Kommu, Kamran Ahmed, Benjamin Challacombe, Prokar Dasgupta, Mohammed Shamim Khan, STILUS Academic Research Group (SARG)

Chapter 4 **Prostate Stones 29**
Hikmet Köseoğlu

Chapter 5 **Ureteric Function and Upper Urinary Tract Urodynamics in Patients with Stones in Kidney and Ureter 37**
Mudraya Irina and Khodyreva Lubov

Chapter 6 **Prevention of Bladder Tumor Recurrence 69**
Shapiro Amos and Ofer N. Gofrit

Chapter 7 **The Emerging Use of Smarthphone apps in Urology 77**
Jonathan Makanjuola and Artaches Zakarian

Preface

Urology is currently the most rapidly expanding surgical superspecialty. The reason for this exponential propulsion of this field, especially over the last two decades, is the dual role of scientific breakthroughs and the successful coupling of engineering and technology for diagnostics and treatment. The role of minimally invasive approaches to surgical extirpation and reconstruction has been unprecedented and paramount. Not only is there rapid development within each substrata of urology but these developments are continuously evolving. This book is the first in a series that explores the current evolving trends in urology. The focus of the book is broad and includes strata of the field including stone disease, telerobotic surgery and surgical simulation. The role of internet based "Apps" are also explored. Some chapters explore leading edge concepts while others capture the evolving trends and future concepts.

Sashi S. Kommu
Urology Centre, Guy's Hospital,
Guy's and St Thomas' NHS Foundation Trust,
London,
UK

1

Telementoring and Telerobotics in Urological Surgery

Yasmin Abu-Ghanem[1], Sarah Wheatstone[2] and Benjamin Challacombe[1]
[1]Guy's and St Thomas NHS Foundation Trust, London,
[2]South London Healthcare NHS Trust, London,
UK

1. Introduction

For decades, doctors have been able to communicate and deliver medical information over long distances and assist their colleagues in remote locations via teleconsultation using a variety of communication modalities.

These long distance forums are better known today as 'Telemedicine'.

At the simplest level, telemedicine is broadly defined as the transfer of electronic medical data (i.e. high resolution images, sounds, live video and patient records) from one location to another [S. K. Dey Biswas, 2002].

By the use of various technologies as the telephone, computers and the internet, communication between physicians in different locations is being held in real-time, and medical information is broadcasted.

Over the past few decades, this transatlantic communication has become more and more common within the medical field, as telemdecine being utilized by a range of specialties and disciplines, especially dermatology [Burg G ,2005].

Despite the rather simple definition, there is no common concurrence on what telemedicine really is; trying to clarify things, the European Commission describe telemedicine as the "rapid access to shared and remote medical expertise by means of telecommunications and information technologies, no matter where the patient or relevant information is", while the American Medical Association (AMA) has defined telemedicine as "medical practice across distance via telecommunications and interactive video technology" [AMA Joint Report, 1994].

Nevertheless, Telemedicine is not a specific procedure or a system; it is a route to convey medical services by merging between the old and the new, the known, conventional medical care with the benefits of current technology, in order to deliver health care globally [Wootton R, 2001].

This technology offers the opportunity to advise local and distanced physicians during patient session and surgeries and by that may proffer better care for the patients.

Moreover, it is also used to connect medically deprived or geographically distant districts, so that less trained on-site physicians can provide health services using this long-distance help.

Less developed countries very often suffer from medical deprivation, starting from the distance to the healthcare centres, to the lack of skilled doctors;

Telemedicine opened the way to healthcare techniques, approaches and medical skills that were not even considered in these districts [WHO 2004, WITSA 2006].

2. Then and now

Doctors have been able to convey medical information across great distances, even before the initial development of telegraphy by Sir Charles Wheatstone in 1837 or the telephone by Alexander Graham Bell in 1875.

In its early manifestation, described in the early 1900, people living in remote areas of Australia used two-way radios, powered by a dynamo driven by a set of bicycle pedals, to communicate with the Royal 'Flying Doctor Service of Australia'.

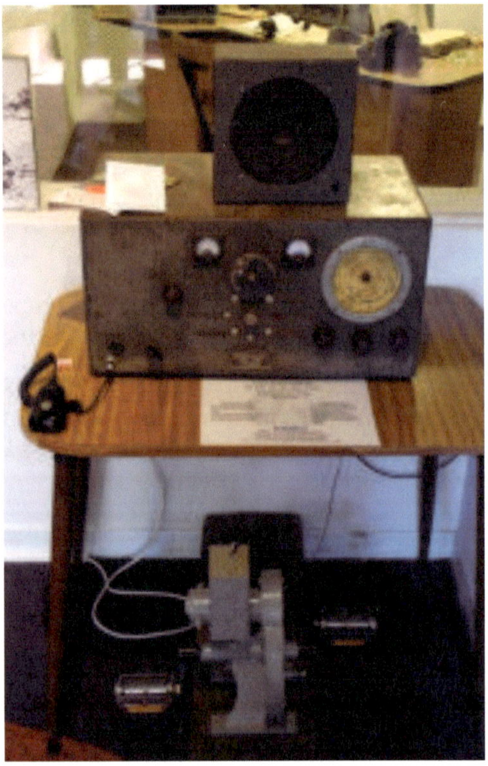

Fig. 1. Traeger pedal-driven radio

The original 1927 Traeger pedal-driven radio receiver at the Royal Flying Doctor Service Station in Alice Springs, Northern Territory, Australia (Challacombe B. et al, 2010).

Other Telemedicine examples date back to the 1930s, when widespread radio communication has just been established. Then it was used to link physicians worldwide and transfer medical information.

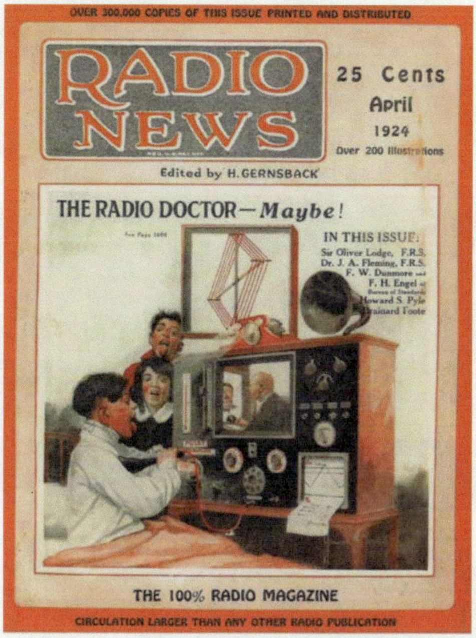

Fig. 2. "The Radio Doctor—Maybe!" Radio News, April 1924

Radio News magazine cover (science magazine of the mid-1920s) predicts the potential progress in telecommunication (radio, telegraph, telephone and television) in medicine ('Radio News', April 1924)

The real development of the telemedicine started by early 1960's, as the National Aeronautics and Space Administration (NASA) used it to deliver physiological parameters from both the spacecraft and the space suits during missions [Bashshur and Lovett, 1977]. Doing so, NASA allowed the following development of satellites communications and telemedicine.

By late 1970's, satellite telemedicine was founded, and paramedics in distant Alaskan and Canadian villages were linked with hospitals in out of reach towns or cities via ATS-6 satellites.

Since the medical world was able to see the benefits of rapid and precise communication over large distances and its potential to aid patients, the concept of 'healing at a distance' has been explored and developed vastly.

Over the last years, it has become part of a growing number of medical specialties such as oncology, pathology, radiology, cardiology, surgery, psychiatry, emergency medicine, nephrology and urology.

3. Telemedicine, looking through the keyhole

Over the last two decades, there has been an ever-increasing number of minimally invasive surgical techniques, also known as the "keyhole procedures"; including laparoscopic and robotically assisted surgery.

This is a modern surgical technique in which operations are performed through small incisions (about 0.5–1.5 cm) as compared to the larger incisions needed in laparotomy.

In order to view the operative field, the laparoscopic surgery uses a video camera that displays the images on TV monitors for enlargement of the surgical elements.

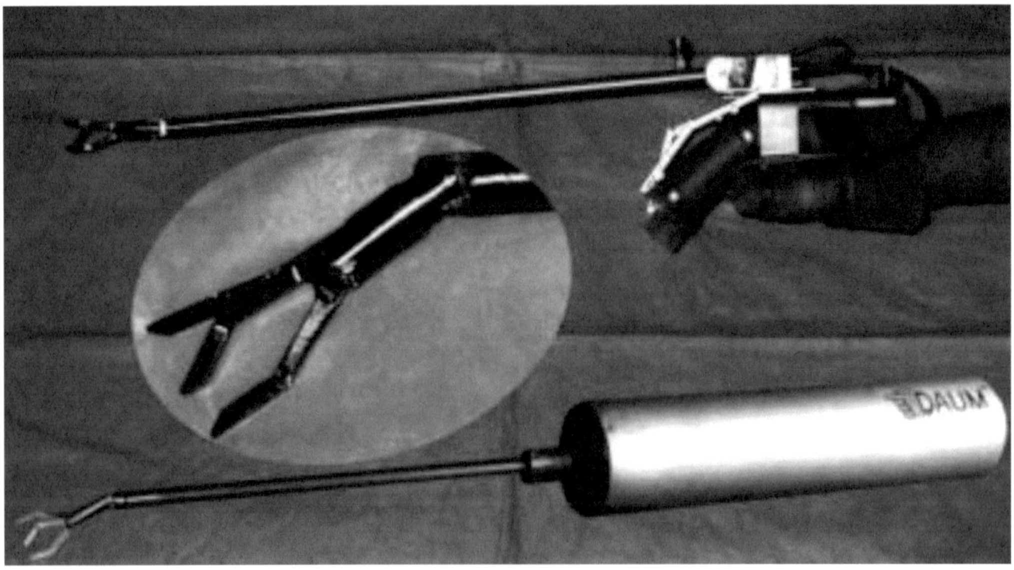

Fig. 3. Laparoscopic instruments, The DAUM EndoHands: Local and remote (Stoianovici D. et al, 2000).

Although these procedures were in evolution for several decades, it was not until the mid1990's that they became acceptable surgical techniques in urology and general surgery. Prior to that, the only specialty performing laparoscopy on a widespread basis was gynecology, mostly for moderately short, simple procedures.

Today, after been proven to produce clinical benefits for countless patients, laparoscopic procedures have advanced to becoming a leading technique in our daily practice.

Minimally invasive surgeries, when performed by experienced surgeons, are favorable for the patients themselves, the hospital and the operating surgeons, with regard to length of hospital stay, return to full activity, and improved cosmetic results [Challacombe B, 2010]. ; Also, they are often more cost-effective than open procedures.

Furthermore, since such surgical procedures are viewed by means of a television monitor they are considered to be ideally suited for the transmission of video images to other sites, and thus, creating a field in which telemedicine techniques can be easily incorporated.

However, although laparoscopic surgery is undoubtedly profitable in terms of patient outcomes, the procedure is more difficult from the surgeon's perception when compared to conventional, open surgery. These procedures are technically demanding, difficult to master and have associated complications that are inversely related to surgeon experience, therefore, having a significant learning curve.

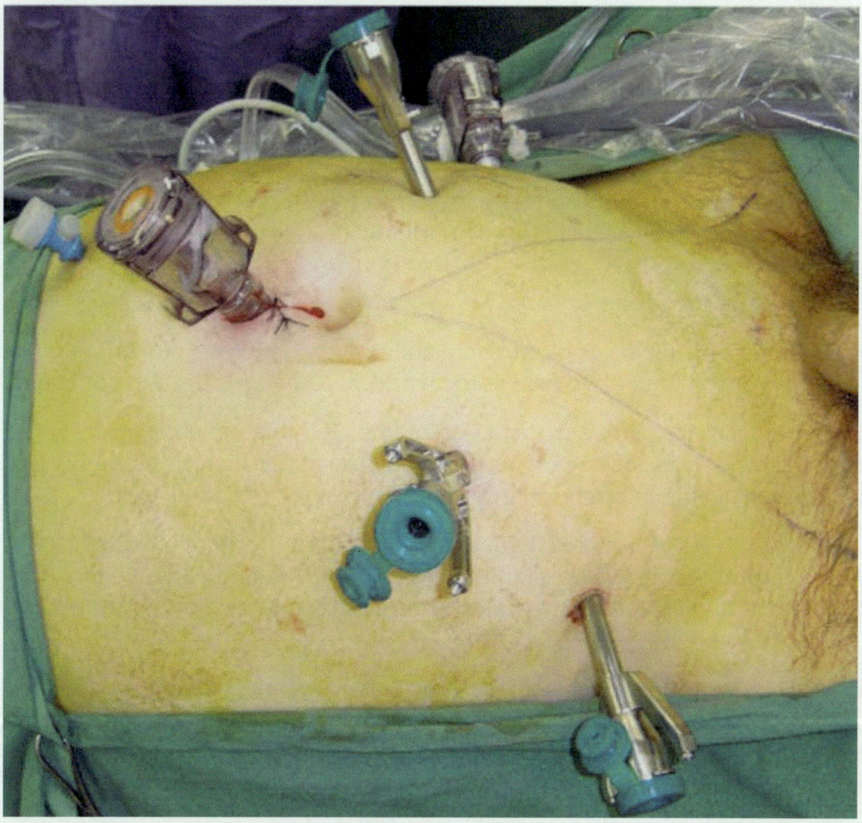

Fig. 4. Minimal Access Surgery Positioning of six ports in a keyhole operation (Van Appledorn S. et al, 2006).

The initial high complication rates associated with minimally invasive surgery and a lack of experienced endoscopic surgeons have raised concerns relating to training and, most importantly, patient safety, consequently, generating a doubt regarding the role of minimally invasive procedures in everyday clinical practice.

However, since the key factor is better training and guidance, it seems that telemedicine may just be the answer to these concerns

By using a real-time video and information transfer, mentoring via telemedicine offers the potential to improve surgeons' skills worldwide and to increase the availability of minimally invasive surgery through video-assisted surgery and through remote instruction.

This long distance guidance, also known as telementoring, may actually answer some of these concerns by allowing better training by closer and tighter guidance.

4. Telementoring

Telesurgical education and mentoring has evolved as an important subset of telemedicine. When applied to surgery, telementoring is used when an experienced surgeon assists or directs another less experienced surgeon who is operating at a distance.

By the usage of two- and three-dimensional, video-based laparoscopic procedures as a platform for real-time transmission, one health care professional can guide, direct, and interact with another, in a different location during an operation or clinical episode.

Communication abilities keep advancing along with technology. These facilities vary from a simple verbal guidance while watching a real-time operation transmitted by video, to indicating target areas on the local monitor screen (telestration), controlling the operative camera, or taking over as the assistant by controlling instruments via a robotic arm.

4.1 Technical considerations

The key point in telemedicine, is offering the ability to bring the encounter to any desk-top, of any provider, at any time, anywhere in the world, at a good picture and audio quality.

A high-speed connection with sufficient bandwidth (the total amount of data sent on the network per second. It usually refers to the maximum application throughput) is required for a proper, high quality telementoring system.

For example, an integrated services digital network (ISDN) connection, with a bandwidth of 384 kB per second (six lines) is required to give sufficient picture quality for precise elucidation by the adviser (although clinical work has been carried out using bandwidths as low as 128 Kb per second [Rosser JC, ,1999].

In terms of connection improvement, the broadband Internet services, as the asymmetric digital subscriber line (ADSL), cable modem service and direct satellite links, have greatly enhanced the telemedicine links, and minimized the delay between the two distant physicians.

A connection delay of less than 250 ms is most likely to be ideal for increased precision, although greater time delays have been shown to be tolerable. Although delays over 500 ms (half a second) are quite noticeable [Fabrizio MD, 2000], surgeons are generally able to compensate for delays of up to 700 ms for remotely performing a surgical task (telesurgery), such as suturing with a robotic device.

Security is one of the main issues to be addressed in terms of clinical data being delivered. In order to ensure it, a VPN ('virtual private network'), is used, a network path or connection that does not allow other connections to or from it.

For the past several years, the potential of telementoring has been illustrated in inaccessible environments. For example, the Johns Hopkins' Urology team who telementored a laparoscopic nephrectomy to Italy, or adrenalectomy, varicocelectomy, renal cyst ablation and radical nephrectomy to countries like Austria, Singapore and Germany [Fabrizio MD,1998; Rodrigues N, 2003].

These early studies have shown that telementoring can significantly shorten the learning curve and decrease the total complication associated with endoscopic surgeons' lack of experience [Challacombe B, 2005].

4.2 Telemedicine in the Robotics era

The next significant advance in the field of surgery and especially in urology was robotic surgical technology, primary used for procedures like radical prostatectomy for localized prostate cancer.

After it has initially been developed by the US department of defence for use in military battlefield applications, robotic technology was taken on for use in human surgical applications.

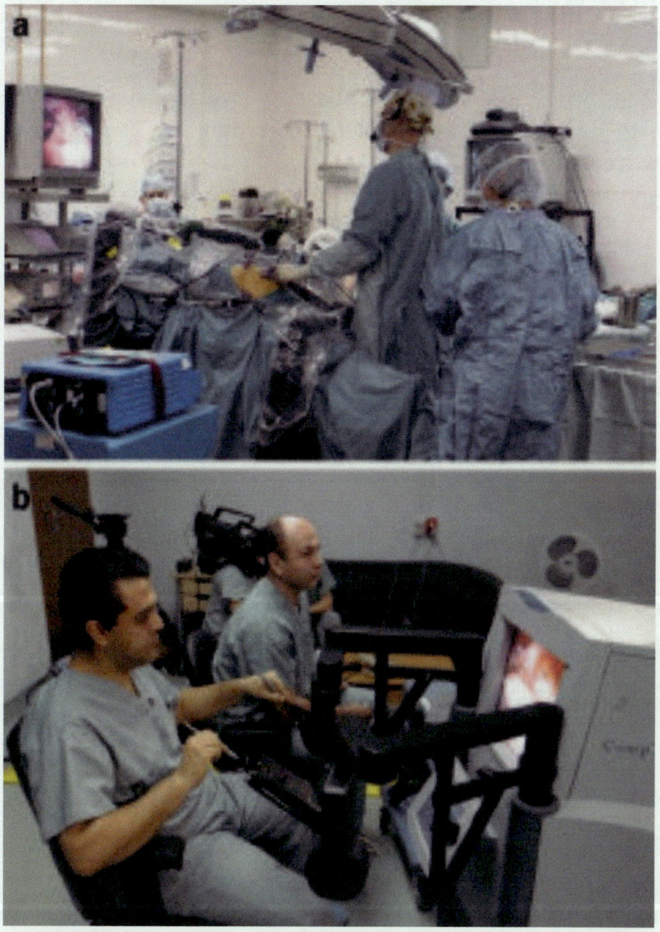

a. Dr. Mehran Anvari at the Zeus TS robotic platform.
b. The remote patient. (Courtesy of M. Anvari,MB, BS, PhD (Challacombe B. et al, 2010).

Fig. 5. Zeus TS robotic platform

Hence, recognizing the potential, around late 90's, two companies introduced their surgical systems almost simultaneously; the Computer Motion, Inc, introduced the Zeus Surgical System and the Intuitive Surgical, Inc, developed its da Vinci Surgical System.

And almost by night, the idea of real telesurgery took one step further, to a real, practical concept.

One of the first examples is the a laparoscopic cholecystectomy, successfully carried out in 2001, using the Zeus robot with the surgeon in New York and the patient in Strasbourg, France [Marescaux J, 2001]. A procedure known today as the 'Lindbergh procedure', named after Charles Lindbergh's first trans-Atlantic flight from New York to Paris.

And by 2005, the da Vinci surgical system had its first public appearance, when Colonel Noah Schenkman of the Walter Reed Army Medical Center performed live nephrectomy on two pigs at the American Telemedicine Association (Washington, DC) [Hanley EJ, 2005].

That operation made history by also being the first to use stereoscopic surgical video streaming, and the first telesurgery over the Internet.

Meanwhile, the Zeus Surgical System was phased out after company takeover, leaving the da Vinci system to thrive around the world, becoming the the current state of the art computer assisted robotic tool today, not only in the field of urology but also in cardiac, gastrointestinal, gynaecologic, paediatric and ENT surgery [Dasgupta P, 2008].

Robotic surgery represents the latest method known for overcoming the obstacles of standard laparoscopy. It trounces various technical challenges by allowing enhanced 3-D visualization, improving dexterity, surgical precision and access, as well as increased range of motion [Ali MR, 2008; Dasgupta P, 2008; Wexner S, 2009].

However, while the potential from robotic procedures seems patently obvious, the learning curve is undeniably steep, therefore requiring lot of guidance and training, making these procedures ideal suited for telementoring.

The robotic surgical system allows the surgeon to transmit data and images to his mentor on line, at any given stage of the operation. The mentor can direct and observe the surgeon is his following steps and indicate appropriate tissue planes or specific lines of incision during the procedure [Challacombe BJ, 2006].

Moreover, in the modern da Vinci Si HD, the system has dual controls, enabling the surgeon to operate while receiving constant feedback from the mentor, who can take over at any point of the operation. That allows the trainee early independence and enhanced training.

Following successful experiments with localized robotic surgeries, the concept was perceived to be extended to remote surgery.

Having its ultimate assemblage for telemedicine, the da Vinci system is often referred to as a "telerobotic" system. In a non robotic operation (open or laparoscopic) the mentor may be remote from the patient, and still advice the leading surgeon, via telecommunicating. However, in order to interfere and control the minimally invasive manipulation, he has to be not only adjacent to the patient, but also scrubbed at all time.

On the other hand, during a robotic procedure, although the mentor will usually be near the patient in the same room, some facilities now have it in a nonscrub area which increases accessibility for the primary surgeon that can now approach easily at any point of the operation and assist, intervene, and carry out a range of operations.

Moreover, a mentor can be present on the patient side as an assistant, and the surgeons are able to switch primary surgeon responsibilities back and forth depending on need. Recently, the da Vinci system has been modified and enabled for use over the Internet as well.

In most general terms, in a telerobotic procedure, the physician is seated at a surgeon console at a distant site, and manipulates remote controls. The joystick or remote control movements are converted into digital signals which travel via the telecommunication network to the robotic system on the patient side. These signals are received by the surgical column and translated from their digital form into movements of the robotic surgical arms within the surgical field (ie, inserted into the patient). The surgeon oversees these movements.

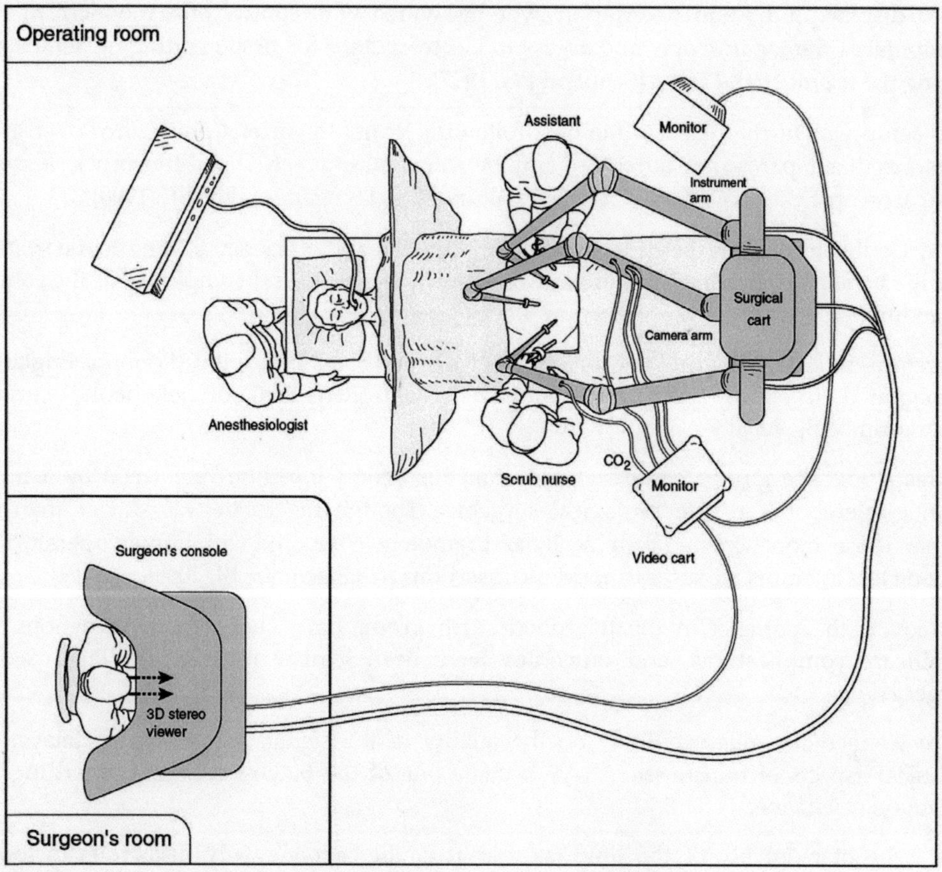

Fig. 6. da Vinci system in operating room (Abbou CC. et al, 2001).

4.3 Telesurgical Telementoring

Since it was first introduced in the early 2000's, the robotic techniques have widely adopted, since it has been shown that they have the advantages of reduced blood loss, reduced pain, shorter inpatient stay and convalescence when compared to open approaches. High volume centres performing these techniques report excellent results with regard to oncological and functional outcomes but there is a lack of level 1 evidence to support their use.

It is likely that robotic prostatectomy using the da Vinci surgical system will be the most common technique in the UK within the next few years and over &)% of radical prostatectomies are performed this way in the United States.

The rapid evolutions of robotics and surgical simulation techniques have facilitated the possibilities of telesurgery with telementoring, telepresence, and telerobotics [Ballantyne GH, 2002].

Therefore, after their initial success with telementoring, the Johns Hopkins Urobotics group established the 'telesurgical mentoring'.

This system increased the telementoring distance to 3.5 miles by integrating the real-time video display, audio and telestration over live video with control of a robotic arm that manipulated the laparoscope, and access to electrocautery for tissue cutting or hemostasis during the telementored cases [Schulam PG, 1997].

This setup was further used in the next following years, in various procedures over great distances, like laparoscopic adrenalectomy between Baltimore, MD and Innsbruck, Austria, or laparoscopic varicocelectomy between Baltimore and Singapore [Lee BR, 1998].

Many doubts have been raised regarding the accuracy and efficiency of the robotic system, and the benefits of telesurgery were outweighed by the costs and complexity of the robotic procedure.

Therefore, in 2002, the Hopkins (Baltimore, MD) and Guy's Hospital (London, England), collaborated to form the first randomized controlled trial of telerobotic surgery [Challacombe BJ, 2003].

In this study, the groups compared percutaneous needle insertion performed by a trans-atlantic telerobotic arm, to urological surgeons. Though the robot was slower than the human it was more accurate both locally and remotely, compared with human operators, as it made less attempts for successful needle insertions [Challacombe BJ, 2005].

Moreover, the patients in the telerobotic arm group have shown no conversions, no significant complications, and outcomes have been similar to standard laparoscopic surgery.

Since telemedicine relays entirely on the quality of the signal, and the time delays, the technical aspects of transmission have become one of the biggest concerns regarding the telerobotic medicine.

The issue of reliability of the link itself, as it could be potentially disastrous to lose a connection at a critical operative stage, has been a major obstacle in the expectance of telemedicine as part of our medical practice.

In order to assess the influence of the technical factor, Challacombe et al. demonstrated that there were no lost signals during the entire procedure. Furthermore, when this group and others investigated the effect of differing time delays on surgical performance, they supported the previous work of Fabrizio et al. who found that errors and task completion times increase only with delays above 500 ms [Anvari N, 2005].

Thus, making it safe to conclude that telerobotic assistance was a significant enabling tool for this type of surgery [Sebajang H, 2006].

5. The future

In the last few decades, medicine has developed alongside a staggering race for technology. Technological Innovations are being vastly used by different medical disciplines, creating the phenomenon we described as telemedicine [Satava RM, 2005].

As technology is being incorporated in the operating room, the complexity of the available surgical equipment continues to advance unabatedly. However, the cost of hardware, software, and the telecommunication link itself begins to fall, and by that, making telesergery and telementoring more accessible, with hopes of becoming a routine application.

Much has been said about the advantages within telemedicine; by telemedicine and telementoring, surgeons can facilitate procedures that would otherwise not even been attempted due to complexity, difficulty, and lack of local surgeon experience.

Using telementoring, surgeons are being guided by their mentors, allowing early independence and reducing learning curves as well as learning time, in new and complex procedures.

Mentors can be "on call" and available at any point, when unexpected operative findings are discovered and aid in any urgent situations owing to their previous experiences.

Surgeons with various expertise can assist and advice their colleges from around the world on their learning, thus, making technically advanced operations available worldwide; developed or underdeveloped countries with remote populations can benefit greatly from telesurgical operating, as a robotic system can be installed locally and an onsite team can be taught how to set up and dock the system [Wynsberghe A, 2008].

In view of the fact that the technology has been available for several years, added to the advantages mentioned above, one would expect that the field of international telementoring will vastly and quickly expend. However, not only that it hardly expanded, for now, it failed to become a bigger part of our medical practice.

Probably the main question asked today, is why; while acknowledging the remarkable benefits technological developments have provided, it is also of great importance to acknowledge their potential harm.

First, is the ethical considerations; one of the ethical dilemmas involves protecting patient confidentiality and privacy while expanding access to information. An electronic communication that includes delivery of sensitive medical data may cause the principles of autonomy and confidentiality to be inadvertently violated [Yeo CJ, 2003].

Although using the VPN, access computerised medical information recorded via the telecommunications network can potentially be compromised and subsequent interruption as honest mistakes, or even deliberate hacking may accrue during telesurgical procedures, which could result in highly sensitive and confidential medical information being shared by basically anyone who could access it.

Another ethical dilemma is the dehumanizing of the patient or reducing it to an object [Wynsberghe A, 2008]. The unconventional long-distance or online consultations practised in telemedicine render it difficult to define the patient-physician relationship.

Many believe that minimizing distances and overseas consultations may actually jeopardise the physician patient relationship. In many of the international cases, a physician may find him self treating a patient he never examined or communicated with, or even met before.

It is clear that every physician has an ethical obligation to his patient; however, it is impossible to determine whether the physician has treated the patient to the best of his capability, and thus decide whether values as integrity and competence, have been strictly held.

Nevertheless, the question whether a patient has to be examined by a certain physician in order to be treated by him should not be related merely to telemedicine; many physician give consultation via the phone or different medical website, without having any knowledge about the patient, apart from what it chose to present.

Another issue that should be addresses, is the differences in both software and hardware capabilities between individual countries.

The cost of buying and installing a high-quality telecommunication system stands, to this date, at approximately $20,000. In hard-wired systems (ie, ISDN) it would be logical for the local center to pay for the telesurgical link, but this may financially prohibit exactly the smaller remote medical centers that stand to benefit most from such systems.

Thirdly, while operating via international telerobotic surgery, a European surgeon may mentor and guide another physician from everywhere around the world. However, to this date, medical qualifications from the European Union are not recognized from the United States and vice versa, therefore, advising to a college overseas who even has his own country specific medical cover may actually raise some ethical and legal issues.

Hence, special arrangements would need to be in place for patient responsibility, and the remote surgeon would have to take liability for the perioperative welfare of patients.

In conclusion, the increasing reliance on computers and information technology in has opened a new window of opportunities to access to medical knowledge and expertise worldwide, simultaneously to cutting costs and increasing efficiency.

From its early examples in early 1900, to the telerobotic era, telemedicine has proven to be efficient in improving availability of selected basic, intermediate and advanced medical facilities, improving diagnoses of diseases due to availability of specialist opinions, convalescing learning curves of advanced and complicated procedures, increased utilization of specialists and in assisting physicians and patients world wide and even reduction the urban migration from villages to major cities due to better medicare.

Therefore, thought ethical, technical and financial issues should be addressed throatily, it is very difficult to comprehend why telecounselling and mentioning has not yet become a major part of our clinical and practical everyday life.

There is no obvious reason why a surgeon should experience difficulties during their learning and hold-up their chance of independence, instead of just taking the opportunity to be instructed by an experienced colleague wherever they are located.

In the future, telemedicine may remedy the uneven geographic distribution of healthcare resources [Challacome BJ, 2006]. It can also address the significant discrepancies in the quality of care available to members of different economic classes [Schulam PG, 1997].

6. References

[1] Abbou CC, Hoznek A, Salomon L, Olsson LE, Lobontiu A, Saint F, Cicco A, Antiphon P, Chopin D (2001). Laparoscopic radical prostatectomy with a remote controlled robot. *J Urol.* 2001 Jun;165(6 Pt 1):1964-6.

[2] Ali MR, Loggins JP, Fuller WD, Miller BE, Hasser CJ, Yellowlees P, Vidovszky TJ, Rasmussen JJ, Pierce J. (2008). 3-D telestration: a teaching tool for robotic surgery. *J Laparoendosc Adv Surg Tech A*. 2008 Feb;18(1):107-12.

[3] Annual Meeting of the American Medical Association (AMA) 1994 ;available <http://www.ama-assn.org/ama/pub/about-ama/our-people/ama-councils/council-science-public-health/reports/19941998-reports.page>

[4] Anvari M, McKinley C, Stein H. (2005). Establishment of the world's first telerobotic remote surgical service for provision of advanced laparoscopic surgery in a rural community. *Ann Surg*. 2005, 241:460–464.

[5] Ballantyne GH. (2002). Robotic surgery, telerobotic surgery, telepresence, and telementoring. Review of early clinical results. *Surg Endosc*. 2002 Oct;16(10):1389-402. Epub 2002 Jul 29.

[6] Bashshur R, Lovett J. (1977). Assessment of telemedicine: results of the initial experience. *Aviat Space Environ Med*. 1977 Jan;48(1):65-70.

[7] Burg G, Hasse U and Cipolat C. (2005). Teledermatology: Just cool or a real tool? *Dermatology*, 2005;210(2):169-73.

[8] Challacombe BJ. (2003). Trans-oceanic telerobotic surgery. *BJU Int* 92: 678–680

[9] Challacombe B, Kandaswamy R, Dasgupta P, Mamode N (2005). Telementoring facilitates independent hand-assisted laparoscopic living donor nephrectomy. *Transplant Proc*. 2005, 37:613–616.

[10] Challacombe B, Patriciu A, Glass J (2005). A randomized controlled trial of human versus robotic and telerobotic access to the kidney as the first step in percutaneous nephrolithotomy. *Comput Aided Surg*. 2005, 10:165–171.

[11] Challacome BJ, Murphy D, Shah N (2006).Trans-atlantic telerobotic watching using the da Vinci Surgical System. *J Endourol*. 2006, 20:A229.

[12] Challacombe B, Wheatstone S. (2010). Telementoring and telerobotics in urological surgery. *Curr Urol Rep*. 2010 Feb;11(1):22-8.

[13] Dasgupta P. (2008). Robotics in urology.*Int J Med Robot*. 2008 Mar;4(1):1-2.

[14] Dey Biswas S. K.; Guest Lecture delivered at BIC Workshop, JBTDRC, Nov. 2002.

[15] Fabrizio MD, Lee BR, Chan DY. (2000). Effect of time delay on surgical performance during telesurgical manipulation. *J Endourol*. 2000, 14:133–138.

[16] Hanley EJ, Miller BE, Herman BC. (2005). Stereoscopic robotic surgical telementoring: feasibility and future applications. Presented at the 10th Annual American Telemedicine Association. Denver, Colorado; April 17, 2005.

[17] Lee BR. (1998) International surgical telementoring: our initial experience. *Stud Health Technol Inform* 50: 41–47

[18] Marescaux J, Leroy J, Gagner M (2001). Transatlantic robotassisted telesurgery. *Nature*. 2001, 413:379–380.

[19] 'Radio News' magazine, April 1924.

[20] Rodrigues Netto N Jr, Mitre AI, Lima SV. (2003). Telementoring between Brazil and the United States: initial experience. *J Endourol. 2003* 17:217–220.

[21] Rosser JC Jr, Bell RL, Harnett B.(1999). Use of mobile lowbandwidth telemedical techniques for extreme telemedicine applications. *J Am Coll Surg*. 1999, 189:397–404.

[22] Satava RM. (2004).Future trends in the design and application of surgical robots. *Semin Laparosc Surg* 2004, 11:129–135.

[23] Schulam PG, Docimo SG, Saleh W. (1997). Telesurgical mentoring. Initial clinical experience. *Surg Endosc* 1997, 11:1001–1005.
[24] Sebajang H, Trudeau P, Dougall A. (2006).The role of telementoring and telerobotic assistance in the provision of laparoscopic colorectal surgery in rural areas. *Surg Endosc.* 2006, 20:1389–1393.
[25] Stoianovici D.(2000). Robotic surgery. *World J Urol.* 2000 Sep;18(4):289-95.
[26] Van Appledorn S, Bouchier-Hayes D, Agarwal D, Costello AJ. (2006). Robotic laparoscopic radical prostatectomy: setup and procedural techniques after 150 cases. *Urology.* 2006 Feb;67(2):364-7.
[27] vanWynsberghe A, Gastmans C: Telesurgery. (2008). an ethical appraisal. J Med Ethics 2008, 34:e22.
[28] Wexner SD, Bergamaschi R, Lacy A, Udo J, Brölmann H, Kennedy RH, John H (2009). The current status of robotic pelvic surgery: results of a multinational interdisciplinary consensus conference. *Surg Endosc.* 2009 Feb;23(2):438-43. Epub 2008 Nov 27.
[29] Wootton R. (2001). Recent advances: Telemedicine. *BMJ.* 2001 Sep 8;323(7312):557-60.
[30] World Health Organisation (WHO), Department of Essential Health Technologies: 'Taking basic health solutions to countries': Strategy 2004-2007 'eHealth for Healthcare Delivery' <http://www.who.int/eht/en/eHealtwfph_HCD.pdf>.
[31] World Information Technology and Services Alliance (WITSA) (2006) 'Health Care and Information and Communications Technologies: Challenges and Opportunities' <http://www.witsa.org/papers/WITSA-HIT-final.pdf>.
[32] Yeo CJ. (2003). Ethical dilemmas of the practice of medicine in the information technology age. *Singapore Med J.* 2003 Mar;44(3):141-4.
[33] Van Appledorn S, Bouchier-Hayes D, Agarwal D, Costello AJ. (2006). Robotic laparoscopic radical prostatectomy: setup and procedural techniques after 150 cases. *Urology.* 2006 Feb;67(2):364-7.

2

Febrile Urinary Tract Infections in Children Less Than 2 Years of Age

Pavel Geier and Janusz Feber
Division of Nephrology, Department of Pediatrics, Children's Hospital of Eastern Ontario, Ottawa, Canada

1. Introduction

Urinary tract infection (UTI) is a common disease in children. In older children the clinical symptoms, diagnostic approach and treatment are similar to adults, whereas infants and neonates present with less specific symptoms. Children post renal transplantation/on immunosuppressive medication may also present with atypical symptoms. Therefore in this chapter we will focus on acute febrile urinary tract infections in young children (aged 2 months to 2 years) and in children post renal transplantation (Tx).

2. Definition

Based on clinical symptoms, UTI's can be divided into three different groups: asymptomatic bacteriuria (ABU), lower UTI (cystitis) and acute pyelonephritis (AP). AP is an infection of the kidney parenchyma and is the most severe form of UTI. In high risk populations (young children, Tx recipients) the AP can cause significant permanent kidney damage resulting in kidney function impairment (Rintaro Mori et al. 2007; Silva et al. 2010; Ramlakhan et al. 2011).

3. Epidemiology

The exact prevalence of UTI's is difficult to assess due to heterogeneity of studies, which includes children of variable ages and genders. The prevalence of UTI's among febrile young children presenting to the emergency department varies between 3.3 and 5.3% (Hoberman et al. 1993; Shaw et al. 1998).

In contrast, the prevalence of febrile UTI in patients post Tx is much higher reaching 15-33% (John & Kemper 2009).

4. Clinical symptoms

High-grade fever is a common symptom of AP. Loin pain, dysuria and urinary frequency may be present, but in young children these symptoms are difficult to discern. Young children can present with only non specific symptoms such as irritability, vomiting, diarrhea and failure to thrive (Clark et al. 2010).

In young children a high grade fever (> 38°C) was found in 83% of patients diagnosed with AP, followed by poor feeding (28%), diarrhea (25%) and failure to thrive (15%) (Kanellopoulos et al. 2006). In children post Tx the most common clinical symptoms are fever, malaise, graft pain and impaired kidney function (John & Kemper 2009).

5. Diagnosis

An early and accurate diagnosis of AP in young children is very important but can be difficult. Delayed diagnosis and/or inadequate treatment of AP may increase the risk of possible permanent kidney damage (Fernández-Menéndez et al. 2003). On the other hand, a false diagnosis of AP may lead to invasive diagnostic imaging and unnecessary treatment without any benefit to the patient (Anon 1999).

The diagnosis of AP is based on a positive urine culture (Mori et al. 2007; Anon 1999); therefore it is crucial to obtain a reliable urine sample for microbiology. The clean-catch urine sample (midstream urine) is appropriate in toilet-trained children, but may be difficult in younger children. In these patients, reliable urine samples can be obtained either by urine catheter or by suprapubic aspiration (SPA). However, both these methods are invasive and should be performed by skilled personnel (Clark et al. 2010). Therefore, an individualized or stepwise approach is recommended. If a child with symptoms suggesting AP is septic and requires immediate antibiotic treatment, the bladder catheterization or SPA is necessary. If however the patient with symptoms of UTI is not severely sick, a urine sample can be obtained by the most convenient method (for example adhesive urine bag) and sent for urinalysis and microscopy. If this urine sample is negative for leukocyte and nitrites, the likelihood of UTI is low (Mori et al. 2010; Ramlakhan et al. 2011); if however leucocytes and/nitrites are detected, a second urine sample should be obtained by a bladder catheter or SPA and sent for urine culture.

Urine culture is considered positive if it grows ≥ 10^7 colony forming units (CFU) of one organism per liter of urine obtained by catheter or ≥ 10^8 CFU in mid-stream urine. Any quantity of a single organism in the urine obtained by SPA is considered a positive urine culture. The diagnosis of AP is usually based on a positive urine culture, high-grade fever, increased white blood cell count with a shift to the left and/or an elevated C-reactive protein.

While these traditional tests suggest renal parenchymal involvement caused by the UTI, the extent and severity of parenchymal lesion/dysfunction is difficult to prove. Recently, serum procalcitonin level has emerged as a marker of parenchymal damage in UTI's (Leroy & Gervaix 2011; Bressan et al. 2009).

The dimercapto-succinic acid (DMSA) isotope exam has been considered as the gold standard to document renal parenchymal inflammation if performed within the first week of symptoms. This investigation is not performed routinely in every patient, but may be helpful in cases in which the diagnosis cannot be established based on urine culture, clinical and laboratory markers (for example a negative urine culture in children who were started on antibiotics before the urine sample was obtained)(Jaksic et al. 2010).

The most predominant bacteria type causing AP in children is Escherichia coli. In the recent study from UK, E.coli caused 92% of acute UTI's in children younger than five years, followed by Proteus (3%) and Pseudomonas (2%)(Chakupurakal et al. 2010). In transplant patients, E coli is the cause of UTI's in only 21-71 % of patients followed by Enterococcus sp (15-33%) and Pseudomonas aeruginosa (4-15%) (John & Kemper 2009).

6. Treatment

The choice of antibiotics for the treatment of AP should be done with respect to local resistance patterns. E. coli, the most common bacteria causing UTI's in children, is usually susceptible to cephalosporins of the third generation or amoxicillin/clavulanate (Hodson et al. 2007). Recently published randomized controlled trials have shown that oral antibiotics are as effective as I.V. antibiotics in the treatment of AP (Pohl 2007; Hodson et al. 2007). I.V. treatment can be limited to children with persistent vomiting or who present seriously unwell; children can then be switched to oral antibiotics as soon as the clinical status allows. Antibiotic treatment should be started as soon as a reliable urine sample is sent for culture. The optimal duration of antibiotic therapy remains a matter of debate; at least 10 days are recommended for treatment of AP (Hodson et al. 2007).

Long-term antibiotic prophylaxis after the first febrile uncomplicated UTI has been a matter of heated discussion among pediatricians/nephrologists and urologists. Most authors agree that it is generally not recommended in children with normal renal ultrasound findings, as there is a lack of evidence of any benefit of prophylaxis for the prevention of relapses of symptomatic UTI and development of new kidney damage (Williams et al. 2006; Montini & Hewitt 2009). However, a recently published randomized controlled trial (RCT) showed that, in a subgroup of girls with high grade (III-IV) vesicoureteric reflux (VUR), those patients who received long term antibiotic prophylaxis, developed new scarring less often (Brandström et al. 2010). Another RCT showed a mild reduction in UTI recurrence in the prophylactic group and authors concluded that "it would be reasonable for clinicians to recommend the use of trimethoprim–sulfamethoxazole in children who are at high risk for infection or whose index infection was severe. Established risk factors for urinary tract infection are female gender, vesicoureteral reflux and particularly, recurrent urinary tract infection"(Craig et al. 2009). In view of these controversial opinions on antibiotic prophalaxis, it seems reasonable to consider prophylaxis on an individual basis, especially in girls.

The antibiotic of choice for long-term prophylaxis is trimethoprim/sulfamethoxazole; the usual dose is 2 mg/kg of trimethoprim (TMP) given at bedtime. TMP alone can be used as an alternative, as its efficacy is the same as the combined TMP/sulfamethoxazole, but the TMP has less adverse effects (Nguyen et al. 2010). In children who do not tolerate or who develop resistance to TMP/ sulfamethoxazone, cephalosporins of the first or second generation (cefalexin, cefadroxil at dose of 10 mg/kg/per day (Saadeh & Mattoo 2011)) or nitrofurantoin (1 mg/kg/day) can be considered.

7. Imaging after the first febrile UTI

The American Academy of Pediatrics recommends that children between the ages of 2 months and 2 years undergo renal ultrasound (US) and voiding cystouretrography (VCUG) after the first febrile UTI (Anon 1999). This recommendation was based on the assumption that this imaging would allow the detection of children with obstructive uropathy and VUR who are at risk of recurrent UTI's and, if untreated, at risk of permanent renal damage.

The widespread use of antenatal US in recent decades has significantly changed the pattern of congenital uropathies. Nowadays, the most severe cases are diagnosed antenatally and appropriate investigation and treatment is done during the neonatal period before these children develop a UTI. It is therefore questionable whether VCUG is really necessary in all children after their first febrile UTI. Recently published meta-analysis showed that a) the VUR was detected in 25% of children with the first febrile UTI, but only 2.5% of children had a high grade VUR (grade IV and V); b) the risk of renal scarring increases with the severity/grade of VUR (Shaikh et al. 2010). One may therefore assume that only patients with high grade VUR would be at risk for scarring. However, renal scars can develop even without the presence of VUR (Moorthy et al. 2005). It is therefore difficult to prove whether the scar is a result of UTI alone, or VUR or both. Overall, permanent renal scars have been found in 15% of children after the first UTI (Shaikh et al. 2010).

Other studies in children with normal antenatal US report the incidence of renal scarring ranging between 4.5 to 16.9% (Garin et al. 2006; Hoberman et al. 2003; Shaikh et al. 2010).

In view of the relatively high percentage of renal scarring post UTI, not necessarily related to the presence of VUR, it seems more important to focus on the detection of renal parenchymal damage, rather than detecting VUR at the time of the first UTI. Some authors therefore suggest to perform US and DMSA scans to detect renal scars and limit the VCUG in patients with evidence of renal scarring (Hardy & Austin 2008). The advantage of this so-called top-down approach is that no patient with permanent kidney damage secondary to febrile UTI is missed and that the VCUG is indicated less often.

In conclusion, UTI's are relatively frequent in young children less than 2 years of age and in children post Tx, can present diagnostic dilemmas and may lead to kidney parenchymal damage if untreated or not treated properly in a timely fashion.

8. References

Anon, 1999. Practice parameter: the diagnosis, treatment, and evaluation of the initial urinary tract infection in febrile infants and young children. American Academy of Pediatrics. Committee on Quality Improvement. Subcommittee on Urinary Tract Infection. *PEDIATRICS*, 103(4 Pt 1), pp.843–852.

Brandström, P. et al., 2010. The Swedish reflux trial in children: IV. Renal damage. *The Journal of Urology*, 184(1), pp.292–297.

Bressan, S. et al., 2009. Procalcitonin as a predictor of renal scarring in infants and young children. *Pediatric Nephrology*, 24(6), pp.1199–1204.

Chakupurakal, R. et al., 2010. Urinary tract pathogens and resistance pattern. *Journal of clinical pathology*, 63(7), pp.652–654.

Clark, C.J., Kennedy, W.A. & Shortliffe, L.D., 2010. Urinary tract infection in children: when to worry. *The Urologic clinics of North America*, 37(2), pp.229–241.

Craig, J.C. et al., 2009. Antibiotic prophylaxis and recurrent urinary tract infection in children. *The New England journal of medicine*, 361(18), pp.1748–1759.

Fernández-Menéndez, J.M. et al., 2003. Risk factors in the development of early technetium-99m dimercaptosuccinic acid renal scintigraphy lesions during first urinary tract infection in children. *Acta paediatrica*, 92(1), pp.21–26.

Garin, E.H. et al., 2006. Clinical significance of primary vesicoureteral reflux and urinary antibiotic prophylaxis after acute pyelonephritis: a multicenter, randomized, controlled study. *PEDIATRICS*, 117(3), pp.626–632.

Hardy, R.D. & Austin, J.C., 2008. DMSA renal scans and the top-down approach to urinary tract infection. *The Pediatric infectious disease journal*, 27(5), pp.476–477.

Hoberman, Alejandro et al., 2003. Imaging studies after a first febrile urinary tract infection in young children. *The New England journal of medicine*, 348(3), pp.195–202.

Hoberman, A et al., 1993. Prevalence of urinary tract infection in febrile infants. *The Journal of pediatrics*, 123(1), pp.17–23.

Hodson, E.M., Willis, N.S. & Craig, J.C., 2007. Antibiotics for acute pyelonephritis in children. *Cochrane database of systematic reviews (Online)*, (4), p.CD003772.

Jaksic, E. et al., 2010. Diagnostic role of initial renal cortical scintigraphy in children with the first episode of acute pyelonephritis. *Annals of Nuclear Medicine*, 25(1), pp.37–43.

John, U. & Kemper, M.J., 2009. Urinary tract infections in children after renal transplantation. *Pediatric Nephrology*, 24(6), pp.1129–1136.

Kanellopoulos, T.A. et al., 2006. First urinary tract infection in neonates, infants and young children: a comparative study. *Pediatric nephrology (Berlin, Germany)*, 21(8), pp.1131–1137.

Leroy, S. & Gervaix, A., 2011. Procalcitonin: a key marker in children with urinary tract infection. *Advances in Urology*, 2011, p.397618.

Montini, G. & Hewitt, I., 2009. Urinary tract infections: to prophylaxis or not to prophylaxis? *Pediatric Nephrology*, 24(9), pp.1605–1609.

Moorthy, I. et al., 2005. The presence of vesicoureteric reflux does not identify a population at risk for renal scarring following a first urinary tract infection. *Archives of disease in childhood*, 90(7), pp.733–736.

Mori, Rintaro, Lakhanpaul, M. & Verrier-Jones, K., 2007. Diagnosis and management of urinary tract infection in children: summary of NICE guidance. *BMJ (Clinical research ed)*, 335(7616), pp.395–397.

Mori, R et al., 2010. Diagnostic performance of urine dipstick testing in children with suspected UTI: a systematic review of relationship with age and comparison with microscopy. *Acta paediatrica (Oslo, Norway : 1992)*, 99(4), pp.581–584.

Nguyen, H.T. et al., 2010. Trimethoprim In Vitro Antibacterial Activity is Not Increased by Adding Sulfamethoxazole for Pediatric Escherichia coli Urinary Tract Infection. *JURO*, 184(1), pp.305–310.

Pohl, A., 2007. Modes of administration of antibiotics for symptomatic severe urinary tract infections. *Cochrane database of systematic reviews (Online)*, (4), p.CD003237.

Ramlakhan, S.L., Burke, D.P. & Goldman, R.S., 2011. Dipstick urinalysis for the emergency department evaluation of urinary tract infections in infants aged less than 2 years. *European journal of emergency medicine* 18(4), pp. 221-4.

Saadeh, S.A. & Mattoo, T.K., 2011. Managing urinary tract infections. *Pediatric Nephrology* 26(11), pp.1967-76.

Shaikh, N. et al., 2010. Risk of renal scarring in children with a first urinary tract infection: a systematic review. *PEDIATRICS*, 126(6), pp.1084–1091.

Shaw, K.N. et al., 1998. Prevalence of urinary tract infection in febrile young children in the emergency department. *PEDIATRICS*, 102(2), p.e16.

Silva, A. et al., 2010. Risk factors for urinary tract infection after renal transplantation and its impact on graft function in children and young adults. *The Journal of Urology*, 184(4), pp.1462–1467.

Williams, G.J. et al., 2006. Long-term antibiotics for preventing recurrent urinary tract infection in children. *Cochrane database of systematic reviews (Online)*, 3, p.CD001534.

3

Evolving Role of Simulators and Training in Robotic Urological Surgery

Sashi S. Kommu[1], Kamran Ahmed, Benjamin Challacombe, Prokar Dasgupta, Mohammed Shamim Khan, STILUS Academic Research Group (SARG)

MRC Centre for Transplantation, King's College London, King's Health Partners, Department of Urology, Guy's Hospital Simulation and Interactive Learning (SaIL) Centre, Guy's & St Thomas NHS Foundation Trust Department of Urology, London, and STILUS Academic Research Group (SARG), London, UK

1. Introduction

The evolution of minimally invasive urological extirpative and reconstructive surgery from the conventional laparoscopic approach to the now widely accepted robotic platforms has entered a new phase. The robotic approach is now considered the gold standard across various centres. With the current and near exponential uptake of the robotic platforms, come challenges for both trainers and trainees. Therefore a demand for up to date training and assessment curriculum is increasing. Currently, training in robotics is not globally standardised, centralised or structured.

Training can be at the work place or in a simulated environment. Whereas simulation is not purported to be an alternative, it can supplement and act as an adjunct to the 'real' environment. Like other craft disciplines such as general surgery and interventional radiology, urology is embracing the increasingly effective role in simulation-based training.

This article aims to identify available training modalities for robotics in urology, highlight deficiencies in the current literature and to provide recommendations for training in robotics based on the current evidence.

2. Available training modalities and their effectiveness

Modern urology training encompasses open surgery along with endoscopic, laparoscopic and more recently robotic surgery. As traditional apprenticeship methods has been shown to be useful for open and some laparoscopic cases, whereby the mentor 'holds' the trainee's hand during the learning phase. This has changed with the introduction of the robotic platform. There is wide variation to what is considered as the 'learning curve' for any given robotic surgical procedure. A structured training and mentoring programme can expedite a

---

[1] Corresponding Author

surgeon's progress in a safe and effective manner from preclinical to table side assistant role and finally to the robotic console.

Surgical simulators have proven to improve the performance in laparoscopic suturing techniques [1]. Virtual reality robotic surgical training offers to shorten the learning curve through repeated simulation of tasks without posing the logistical and ethical challenge of using animal models [2]. A virtual reality robotic simulator for the da Vinci system has recently been tested and appears to be promising, with further research being carried out to improve its efficiency [3].

In an American study using preclinical surgical robotic programme with animal model, the learning curve was found to be shortened whilst reducing the set-up and operative time [4]. It allows refinement of surgical technique prior to use in humans. Robotic surgical training system also allows for technical improvement whilst monitoring and reducing errors and allowing evaluation of performance [5]. An earlier study using Zeus robotic surgical system on laparoscopic trainer, showed faster timings for more experienced surgeons [6]. A systematic training approach for robotic prostatectomy with a step by step assessment and progression has been advocated for a safe and proficient training [7].

Robotic surgical training has now been incorporated in structured training programmes [7-9]. With structured training, no significant adverse impact on outcomes was seen for robotic prostatectomy done by urology fellows for over 1800 patients in a high volume centre [8]. Using a robotic surgical simulator (RoSS),'Hands-On Surgical Training (HOST)' software has been developed recently [10]. This prompts and helps in real-time during the procedure along with evaluating performance and progression. The lack of haptic feedback with traditional robotic training and surgery [11], was overcome with the dv-Trainer, a virtual reality simulator for da Vinci Surgical System [12]. Although still being developed, the authors conclude that the haptic feedback, virtual reality and instrumentation all achieved acceptability.

A 5-day mini robotic fellowship with tutorials, lectures, clinical observership, animal and cadaveric training showed 86% participants performing robotic prostatectomies at 3 years [13]. A system of extended-proctorship programme for robotic prostatectomy has been advocated as a part of post-graduate training in a 3-phase curriculum [14]. The first phase consisted of a 2-day robotic training course wherein stepwise instructions on using the da Vinci robot were given, with time to practice camera and clutching navigation. This was combined with tasks on practical skills such as dissection and suturing on a porcine model including nephrectomy and urethrovesical anastomosis. The second phase comprised of assisting the proctor in 5-6 robotic prostatectomies. Finally, more console autonomy was given as the training progressed, eventually with proctors assisting the trainees whilst providing feedback to them. With gradual progression, the steps performed increased from easier steps such as port placement to more complex difficult steps such as urethrovesical anastomosis and performing nerve-sparing technique. Their programme received a rating of 4.2/5 for effectiveness in robotic training skills, with an average of 20 cases performed in phase 3 before practicing independently.

Although the animal model and virtual reality da Vinci training can provide simulation experience, resource limitation and ethical dilemma prevent their widespread use. With robotic surgery continuing to develop and expand, there is an urgent need for investment into other forms of simulators and training, including the use of virtual reality and synthetic models for training.

3. Trainee impact on patient outcomes

With the rapid uptake of robotic urological surgery, the question as to the impact of the learning curve on patient safety, including oncological control, is under scrutiny. Opinion varies amongst expert consensuses.

In a study looking at the pathologic outcomes during the learning curve for robotic-assisted laparoscopic radical prostatectomy, Shah et al. reported their initial experience with 62 patients undergoing robotic-assisted laparoscopic prostatectomy (RALP), focusing on the primary parameter of positive surgical margins [19]. Their study seemed to suggest that RALP could have equal if not better pathologic outcomes compared to open radical prostatectomy even during the initial series of cases. They argued that the learning curve for RALP is shorter than previously thought. They concluded that previous purported concerns with respect to oncological outcomes as a result of lack of tactile feedback were unfounded. Schroeck et al. [20] evaluated the learning curves and perioperative outcomes of an experienced laparoscopic surgeon and his trainees to gain some insight into the question of whether trainees negatively impact on the institutional learning curve for robotic prostatectomy as characterized by operative time, estimated blood loss, and positive surgical margin rate. They concluded that a structured teaching program for RALP is effective and that trainees did not negatively affect the estimated blood loss and positive surgical margin rate. Pruthi et al. sought to evaluate the learning curve of robot-assisted laparoscopic radical cystectomy by evaluating some of the surgical, oncological, and clinical outcomes in our initial experience with 50 consecutive patients [21]. In their series of 50 cases they found that despite the higher blood loss that is observed early in the learning curve, no such compromises were observed with regard to these oncological parameters even early in the experience.

Hong et al. postulated that a definitive RALP "learning curve" has not been defined and that existing learning curves do not account for urologists without prior advanced laparoscopic and robotic skills [22]. They proposed 'an easily evaluable metric' i.e. "oncological experience curve," that could potentially be clinically useful to all urologists performing RALP. They found in their study that the oncological experience curve may be much longer than the previously reported learning curves. They concluded that surgeons should consider whether they can build enough experience to minimize suboptimal oncological outcomes before embarking on or continuing a RALP program. Kwon et al. attempted to prospectively compare outcomes during robotic prostatectomy between surgeons with formal training in either robotic prostatectomy (RALP) or laparoscopic prostatectomy (LRP) [23]. Twelve urologists conducted 286 robotic prostatectomies of which 4 surgeons had formal training in RALP and 8 had formal training in LRP. They prospectively compared surgical and pathologic outcomes between these 2 groups of surgeons. They found that the robot-trained surgeons had 10%-15% shorter procedure times. There was no difference in complication rates. They concluded that formal RALP training may be beneficial for surgical and pathologic outcomes of RALP compared with formal LRP training during the initial implementation of a new robotics program.

Currently, there is no published consensus on overall impact of robotic trainees and/or early learning curve on patient outcomes. There are no well structured studies that correlate the effectiveness of training (real or simulated settings) with patient morbidity or mortality data. The few studies conducted looking at other parameters, seem to suggest that there is no adverse impact. However, most of the studies were conducted in centres of excellence and/or high volume units with seeming dedicated and structured mentoring. More studies are required to stratify the direct impact of trainees on outcomes.

4. Problems with the existing training system and tools

The future of robotic training depends on the acceptance of this technology both at the consumer and provider levels [15]. The past decade has witnessed a rapid increase in robotic surgical procedures in terms of its frequency and innovations. Several structural and organizational queries must be addressed before the acceptability and feasibility of the training methods: First, do the results of the existing methods of training are comparable to the patient outcomes? Second, is the skill training on simulators is transferable to the real settings? Third, do we know whether the learning curve can be reduced with additional training on simulators? Fourth, are the new tools cost effective and will they be acceptable by the trainers and trainees? and finally, what is the educational impact of the simulation based training? Geographical variation in the standards of training is a key factor that can affect national and international recognition of training. For instance, all of the European Union (EU) states have certification programs that are significantly different in terminology, guidelines, training and assessment frequency [16]. This may result in issues such as acceptability and feasibility. The system needs to be harmonized to increase the level of acceptability across various regions (**Figure 1**). The existing literature doesn't look into the psychological aspects of training. Training models such as Ericson theory, Schimdt theory and theory of deliberate practice need to be consulted whilst researching various training tools [17, 18].

5. Future recommendations

In a survey of Residency Training in Laparoscopic and Robotic Surgery Duchenea et al. in 2006 attempted to determine the status of residency training in laparoscopic and robotic surgery in the United States and Canada [24]. A total of 1,188 surveys were sent via the Internet to all 1,056 urology residents and 132 program directors. It was noted that a large number of laparoscopic urological procedures were being performed at training institutions with robotic procedures being performed at just over fifty percent of the facilities. Trainees were participating in most cases but only 38% consider their laparoscopic experience to be satisfactory. The study concluded that there was a need for increased laparoscopic training among residents. It was noted that one way of tackling this is to expand training facilities and increase the number of mentors actively performing and tutoring trainees.

Kommu et al. attempted to delineate a preliminary rank stratification of the top ten indices of the ideal robotic urological training programmes [25]. The trainees were asked to rank the top fifteen indices, in the first instance, which they felt represented the ideal robotic

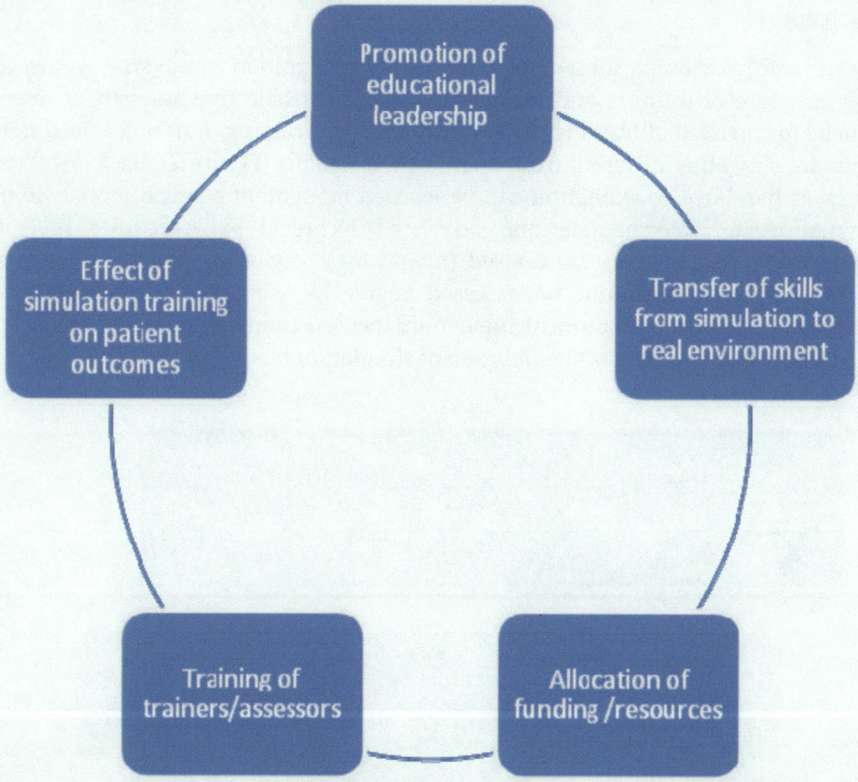

Fig. 1. Issues with the current training system/tools

urological training programmes. One hundred and eighty randomly chosen participants from a database pool of known trainees globally were sent a standard questionnaire by email. The response rate was 84%. The results when tallied in rank order of importance were as follows: 1. Funding and economic constraints, 2. Dry lab training facilities on site, 3. Courses and Meetings, 4. Wet/Animal lab training, 5. Balance and volume of cases, 5. Trainee activity restricted to RAUS only, 6. Mentor/Faculty Resources including feedback facilities, 7. High training time to service provision ratio, 8. Research activity, 9. Attendance by Global Faculty of experts and 10. Streamlining of a dedicated post/job following training period. They concluded that the top ten indices for the ideal Robotic Urological Training Programmes are based on the themes of funding and ease of accessibility to training resources such as courses, hands on training and volume of cases. Knowledge of the identified indices could help training units to further tailor their programmes. They added that their findings could act as a preliminary platform for initiation of subsequent benchmarks for optimal training. Future challenges include establishment of evidence based centralised training programmes that are cost effective. Training of the trainers and assessors is also an important issue that needs considerable research and allocation of funding by the training organisations [26]. Any established training programmes would need general acceptability by the healthcare organisations and trainees. Research to evaluate the effect of simulation training on the outcomes [27].

6. Conclusions

Because of rapidly evolving innovations, increasing recognition of adverse events, changes affecting structure of training and the more demand for objective assessment, there is an urgent need for revision of training programs [27,28,29]. Training in robotics need new set of skills that are altogether different from open technical skills (**Figure 2**). Basic-level technical skills such as hand-eye coordination can be learned on synthetic bench model simulations and animal tissue. Intermediate and advanced technical skills require high fidelity simulations. At a senior level, supervised (mentoring) robotic procedures on patients are crucial to training and should be assessed regularly using objective methods. These objectives can be achieved by introducing a more focused training and assessment pathway, with the further development and validation of simulation models.

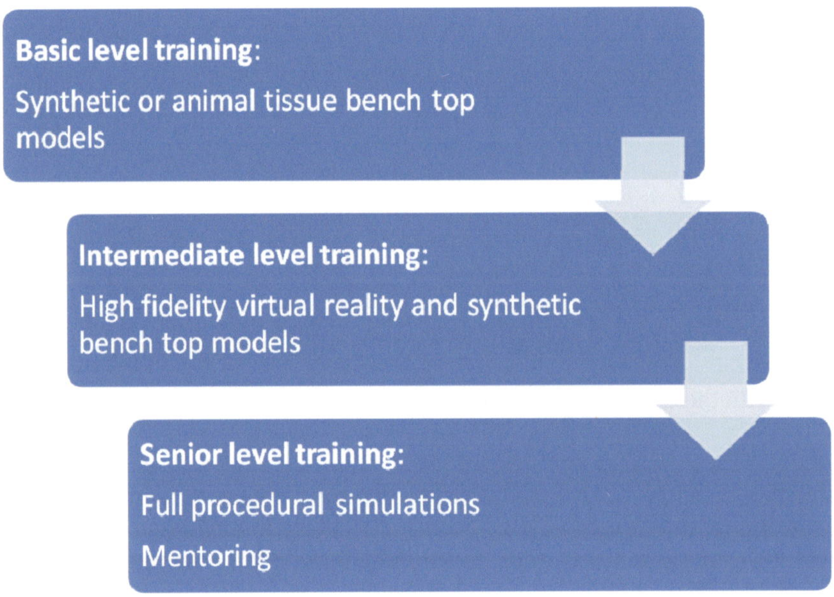

Fig. 2. Recommendations for training curriculum.

7. References

[1] Laguna M P, et al. Construct validity of the chicken model in the simulation of laparoscopic radical prostatectomy suture. J Endourol 2006;20:69-73.
[2] Albani J M, Lee D I. Virtual reality-assisted robotic surgical simulation. J Endourol. 2007 Mar;21(3):285-7.
[3] Katsavelis D, Siu K C et al. Validated robotic laparoscopic training in a virtual-reality environment. Surg Endosc 2009; 23(1):66-73.
[4] Hanly E J, et al. Multiservice laparoscopic surgical training using the daVincisurgical system. American Journal of Surgery 2004 187: 309-315.
[5] Di Lorenzo N, et al. Robotic systems and surgical education. JSLS 2005;9:3-12.
[6] Prasad S M. The effect of robotic assistance on learning curves for basic laparoscopic skills. American Journal of Surgery. 2002: 183: 702-707.

[7] Rashid H H. Robotic surgical education: a systematic approach to training urology residents to perform robotic-assisted laparoscopic radical prostatectomy. Urology 2006 2006 Jul;68(1):75-9.

[8] Link B A. Training of Urologic Oncology Fellows Does Not Adversely Impact Outcomes of Robot-Assisted Laparoscopic Prostatectomy. J Endourol; 2009.

[9] Grover S. Residency training program paradigms for teaching robotic surgical skills to urology residents. Curr Urol Rep. 2010 Mar;11(2):87-92.

[10] Kesavadas T, et al. Efficacy of Robotic surgery simulator (ROSS) for the da Vinci surgical system. www.aua2009/org/abstracts/2009/2271. http://www.bjhcim.co.uk/news/2010/n1006021.htm

[11] van der Meijden O A J, Schijven M P. The value of haptic feedback in conventional and robot-assisted minimal invasive surgery and virtual reality training: a current review. Surg Endosc (2009) 23:1180–1190.

[12] Kenney A P, et al. Validation of the dv-Trainer, A novel virtual reality simulator for robotic surgery. www.aua2009.org/abstracts/2009/2184.

[13] Gamboa AJR, et al. Long-term impact of a robot assisted laparoscopic prostatectomy mini fellowship training program on postgraduate urological practice patterns. J Urol. 2009;181:778 –782.

[14] Mirheydar H, et al. Robotic Surgical Education: a collaborative approach to training postgraduate urologists and endourology fellows. JSLS (2009)13:287–292.

[15] Ahmed K, Khan MS, Vats A, Nagpal K, Priest O, Patel V, Vecht JA, Ashrafian H, Yang GZ, Athanasiou T, Darzi A. Current status of robotic assisted pelvic surgery and future developments. Int J Surg. 2009 Oct;7(5):431-40.

[16] Ahmed K, Ashrafian H, Hanna GB, Darzi A, Athanasiou T. Assessment of specialists in cardiovascular practice. Nat Rev Cardiol. 2009 Oct;6(10):659-67.

[17] Ahmed K, Keeling AN, Fakhry M, Ashrafian H, Aggarwal R, Naughton PA, Darzi A, Cheshire N, Athanasiou T, Hamady M. Role of virtual reality simulation in teaching and assessing technical skills in endovascular intervention. J Vasc Interv Radiol. 2010 Jan;21(1):55-66.

[18] Ericsson KA. The acquisition of expert performance: an introduction to some of the issues. In: Ericsson KA, ed. The road to excellence: the acquisition of expert performance in the arts and sciences, sports, and games. Mahwah, NJ: Lawrence Erlbaum, 1996; 1–50.

[19] Shah A, Okotie OT, Zhao L, Pins MR, Bhalani V, Dalton DP. Pathologic outcomes during the learning curve for robotic-assisted laparoscopic radical prostatectomy. Int Braz J Urol. 2008 Mar-Apr;34(2):159-62; discussion 163.

[20] Schroeck FR, de Sousa CA, Kalman RA, Kalia MS, Pierre SA, Haleblian GE, Sun L, Moul JW, Albala DM. Trainees do not negatively impact the institutional learning curve for robotic prostatectomy as characterized by operative time, estimated blood loss, and positive surgical margin rate. Urology. 2008 Apr;71(4):597-601.

[21] Pruthi RS, Smith A, Wallen EM. Evaluating the learning curve for robot-assisted laparoscopic radical cystectomy. J Endourol. 2008 Nov;22(11):2469-74.

[22] Hong YM, Sutherland DE, Linder B, Engel JD. "Learning curve" may not be enough: assessing the oncological experience curve for robotic radical prostatectomy. J Endourol. 2010 Mar;24(3):473-7.

[23] Kwon EO, Bautista TC, Jung H, Goharderakhshan RZ, Williams SG, Chien GW. Impact of robotic training on surgical and pathologic outcomes during robot-assisted laparoscopic radical prostatectomy. Urology. 2010 Aug;76(2):363-8. Epub 2010 Mar 5.

[24] Duchene DA, Moinzadeh A, Gill IS, Clayman RV, Winfield HN. Survey of residency training in laparoscopic and robotic surgery. J Urol. 2006 Nov;176(5):2158-66; discussion 2167.

[25] Kommu SS, Finnigan T, Cartlidge D, Hamid S, Hashim Z, STILUS Academic Research Group (SARG). Optimal Robotic Urological Training Programmes - Top Ten Indices. Journal of Endourology. Proceedings of the World Congress of Endourology and SWL. Oct 2009.

[26] Ahmed, K., Nagpal, K. & Ashrafian, H. Do we need to train assessors? Med. Educ. 43, 389 (2009).

[27] Ahmed K, Jawad M, Dasgupta P, Darzi A, Athanasiou T, Khan MS. Assessment and maintenance of competence in urology. Nat Rev Urol. 2010 Jul;7(7):403-13.

[28] Gawande AA, Zinner MJ, Studdert DM, Brennan TA (2003) Analysis of errors reported by surgeons at three teaching hospitals. Surgery 133:614–621.

[29] Horton R (2001) The real lessons from Harold Frederick Shipman. Lancet 357:82–83.

4

Prostate Stones

Hikmet Köseoğlu
Baskent University, F.E.B.U.
Turkey

1. Introduction

Being the only exocrine organ located in the midline, the prostate gland is a compound tubuloalveolar exocrine gland of the male reproductive system, locating just below the bladder. The term "prostate" comes (as commonly published) from Greek *prostates*, literally which means "someone who stands before someone or something" that is "president" or "principal" ; however in a recent paper on history of medical terminology it was suggested that in fact the term was originating from Greek *parastates* which means literally "someone who stands next to someone or something" or "companion" and was transformed into *prostates* due to misspelling and misinterpretation [1].

Embryologically, the prostate develops from the endodermal urogenital sinus which is an ambisexual embryonic rudiment. Endodermal urogenital sinus forms the prostate, prostatic urethra and bulbourethral glands in the males and the lower vagina and urethra in the females. The embryonic connective tissue surrounding endodermal urogenital sinus is called urogenital sinus mesenchyme. Under the influence of fetal androgens, epithelial outgrowths from the wall of the urogenital sinus move into the surrounding urogenital sinus mesenchyme forming prostatic glandular structure and the surrounding mesenchyme differentiates into smooth muscle cells and fibroblasts [2]. The secretory epithelium in this compound tubuloalveolar gland structure is mainly pseudostratified with transitional epithelium in the distal regions of the longer ducts. In the prostate gland acini, small round luminal hyaline masses called **corpora amylacea** may be found. With average diameter of 0.25 mm, pink-purple to orange color these masses are believed to be related to epithelial cell desquamation and degeneration. They are composed of bundles of fibrils and containing mainly sulfated glycosaminoglycans [3]. Corpora amylacea are frequently seen in the benign acini of prostates of adult men however, they are rarely seen in prostate carcinoma [4].

2. Prostate stones: Formation and structure

In the literature, sometimes prostatic calculi are classified as either primary /endogenous calculi (developing within the acini of the gland) or secondary/exogenous (upper urinary system stone found in the prostatic urethra). Throughout this chapter, the terms "prostatic calculi" or "prostate stone" refers only to the stones developing within the acini of the gland (primary /endogenous calculi).

The calcification of corpora amylacea within gland acini forms prostate stones. Prostate stones are predominantly found in the cephalic portion of the posterior lobe and in the larger ducts and acini of the lateral lobes of the prostate. Those within the acini are microscopic,while those within the ducts tend to be larger and are visible grossly. Suggested mechanism of the stone formation is the intra-prostatic reflux of urine which causes the deposition of hydroxyapatite crystallites in corpora amylacea and mineralization with calcium, leading to the formation of calculi [5–7]. Obstruction of the acini with calculi causes dilatation of acini and further increase in size of the stone with further precipitation of crystals. As well, the growing calculi itself or together with the inflammatory process, that it may initiate, may occlude other acini causing further stone formation. This way of formation leads to concentric calcification layers in the stone which is clearly seen under scanning electron microscope [8] (Figure 1). Such an occlusion mechanism might be responsible in cases of benign prostate hyperplasia. Observation of prostate stones located in the compressed true prostate adjacent to the adenomatous mass also supports this mechanism [9]. Prostate stones are not infection stones. Major calcium components of prostate stone are calcium phosphate or calcium oxalate, along with carbonate-apatite and hydroxyapatite [7,8,10].

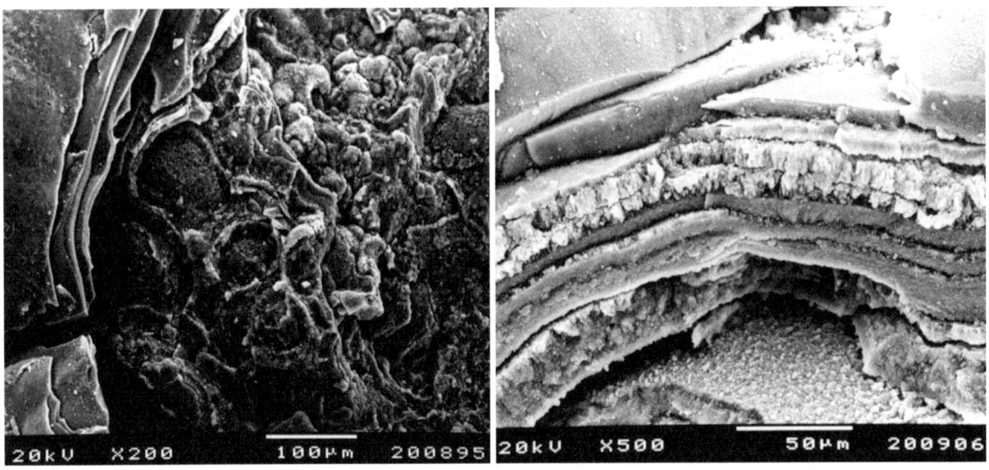

Fig. 1. Concentric calcification layers of prostate stone under scanning electron microscope (Personal archive of Koseoglu H, MD.)

Also, some pathological conditions like alkaptonuria and vitamin D overdose have been reported to cause prostatic calculi [11,12].

Prostate stones were classified structural morphology and mineral composition [13,14] In one older study, stones taken from males with BPH were analyzed with scanning electron microscopy and energy dispersive type X-ray microanalyzer (EDAX) system for structure and element compositions. Mainly, elements of Na, Al, Mg, S, P, Ca and Zn were identified. Stones were classified as type I and type II. Type I prostate stones have lobular surface made up of small spheres containing predominantly of sodium, sulfur, phosphorus, calcium, and zinc. Type II prostate stones have polyfaceted surface composed primarily of calcium phosphate in the form of hydroxyapatite crystals with high peaks of P and Ca [13]. In a rather recent study, the fine structure and mineral components prostate stones were analyzed by scanning electron microscopy, backscattered electron (BSE) imaging, energy-dispersive X-ray (EDX) microanalysis under an SEM and X-ray diffraction [14]. Main element composisiton was Ca,P,Mg, Zn and S. The prostate stones were classified into four groups (I–IV). Group I had the core deposits of calcospherites showing concentric rings and the laminated apatite deposits concentrically around the core. Group II had calcospherite deposits of apatite similar to group I with a rougher concentric formation. Group III similar to group I had the core of calcospherites and concentric laminated structures with wider peripheral region containing calcium oxalates spikes. Gorup IV had the core deposits with small hexahedral structures, identified as whitlockite, surrounded by incompletely concentric laminated bands of apatite. Group I–III were suggested to form from mineralization of corpora amylacea whereas group IV was suggested to form from mineralization of the organic substances, which might be derived from the simple precipitation of prostatic secretion [14].

Other than the crytalline structure of the prostate stones, their protein composition was studied with infrared spectroscopy and high-performance liquid chromatography combined with tandem mass spectrometry (LC/MS/MS) in the prostate stones taken form radical prostatectomy specimen of prostate cancer patients [15]. The predominant crystalline component was also confirmed as calcium phosphate in the form of hydroxyapatite. The most prevalent proteins were lactoferrin, myeloperoxidase, and S100 calcium-binding proteins A8 and A9. Others were multiple proteins found in neutrophil granules. All these proteins act in acute inflammatory pathways. The authors suggested that this may indicate past inflammatory events in the prostate [15].

3. Epidemiology

The data in the literature on the prevalence of prostatic calculi is inconclusive. In a report of postmortem study using microradiographic examination, the intraprostatic calcifications were found to be prevalent as high as 71% [16]. In one study using transrectal ultrasonography prostatic calculi were detected in 198 (40.7%) of the 486 screened man with a mean age of 61.9 +/- 0.4 years (range 29 to 89) [17]. In another study using transrectal ultrasonography prostatic calculi were detected in 799 (51.1%) of 1563 with a younger mean age of 49.5 +/- 5.4 years (range 40 to 59) [18]. Again, in another study done with transrectal ultrasonography prostatic calculi were detected with a similar ratio of 41.77 % [19].

However, in another recent study using transabdominal ultrasonography (TRUS only in 16.83% of cases) the prevalence was found to be low as 7.35% in a screened adult group with a mean age of 40.9 (range 21–50) years [20]. The methodological difference may be a reason of low prevalence. But, in that study the patients were chosen among a population of nonconsecutive 1374 young men that attended the hospital outpatient clinics for several reasons. It is worthy to note that in other studies using transrectal ultrasonography, above mentioned, the study population was chosen from consecutive patients attending urology clinics for routine checkup of PSA and DRE evaluation or with complaints of LUTS or chronic prostatitis/chronic pelvic pain syndrome. That may also be a reason for the high difference between prevalence of the studies.

The youngest patient reported was 4 year old and in that patient the calculi was thought to be related to vitamin D overdose [11].

4. Clinical importance

Prostate stones are generally clinically asymptomatic, when symptomatic the symptoms are generally related to lower urinary tract symptoms [18,19]. The prostatic calculi are mostly found incidentally during diagnostic workup for any urological complaint. In the CT scans, pelvic/transrectal ultrasonography or KUB X-scans they may be found incidentally (Figures 2; 3). They are also frequently encountered during transurethral resection of the prostate [8] (Figure 4). In benign prostatic hyperplasia, prostate stones tend to be located in the compressed true prostate, adjacent to the adenomatous mass [9]. Therefore, during transurethral resection of the prostate, prostate stones are rather observed when the depth of resection increased and thus they act sometimes as a border for prostate capsule during TURP.

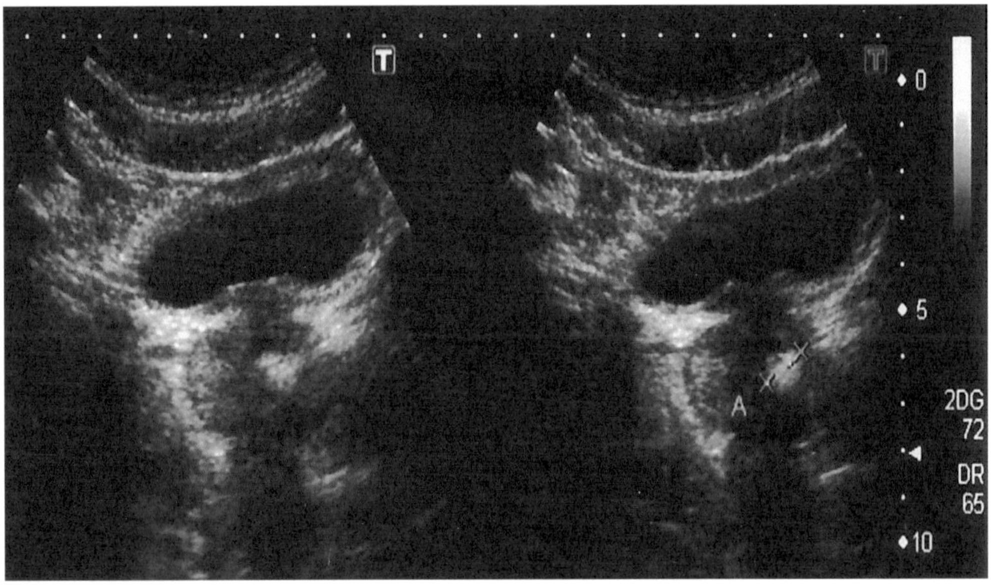

Fig. 2. Pelvic ultrasonography showing prostate stone in the prostate gland (Personal archive of Koseoglu H, MD.)

The presence of large prostatic calculi has been shown to be a significant associated factor of moderate LUTS [18]. In another study, patients with prostate stones were reported to have more severe LUTS and decreased the maximum urinary flow rates compared to patients without prostate stones. However, based on multivariate analyses, prostate stone was not an independent predictive factor of severe LUTS [19]. Rather, older age and larger prostate volume were independent predisposing factors for prostate stone [19].

Larger prostate stones were suggested to have a relation with clinical prostatitis/ chronic pelvic pain syndrome [20]. Histopathological inflammation with varying degrees of severity may accompany prostate stones [8]. However, it is unclear whether inflammation is a cause or the result of calculi formation. The prostatic stones do not raise PSA, which increases with inflammation, indirectly indicating that these calculi do not increase inflammation [17]. On the other hand, intra-prostatic reflux related to prostate stone formation may play a role in the accompanying inflammation of prostate gland. In a study using anti-nanobacterial agent it was shown that prostatic stones diminished 50% ultrasonographically and chronic prostatitis symptom scores were decreased [21]. However, there was no relationship between chronic prostatitis symptom scores and prostatic calculi or level of the histological prostatic inflammation [21].

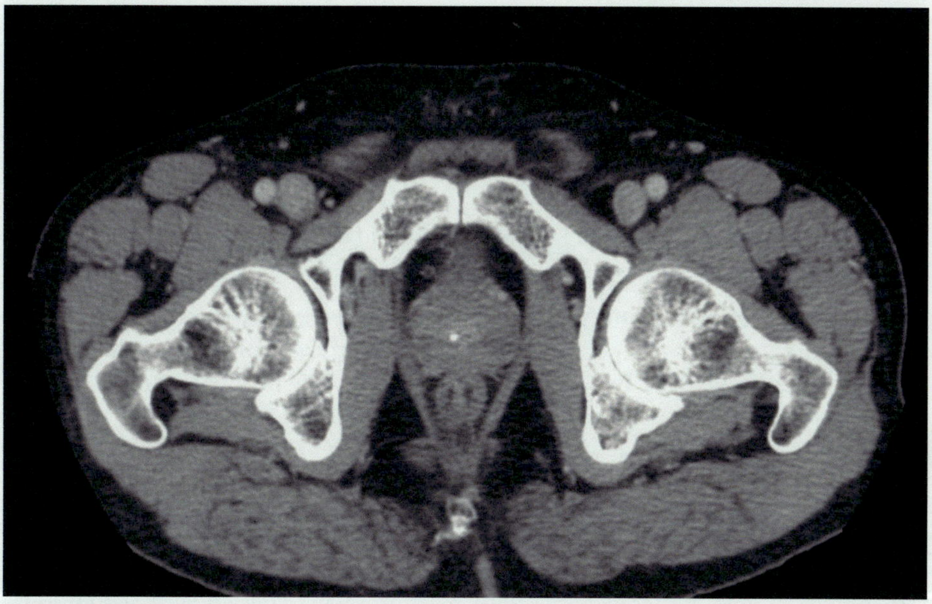

Fig. 3. Pelvic CT scan showing prostate stone in the prostate gland (Personal archive of Koseoglu H, MD.)

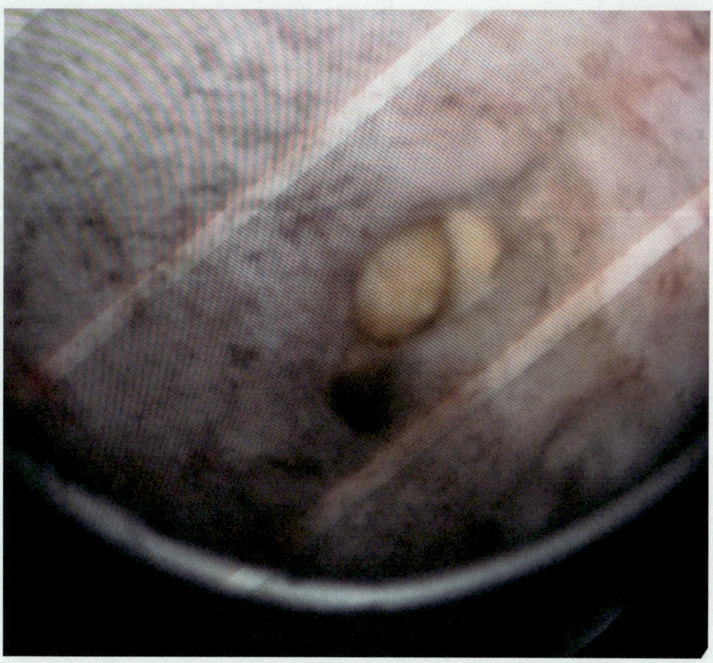

Fig. 4. Prostate stones encountered during TUR-P (Personal archive of Koseoglu H, MD.)

In the literature, there are few case reports related to large prostate stones causing infravesical obstruction [22-27].

No direct or indirect relationship has been reported between prostate stone and prostate cancer. Actually the incidence of corpora amylacea in adenocarcinoma is low [5].

5. Management of prostate stones

Though prostate stones are generally accepted as clinically silent, few cases were reported to have surgical intervention for severe obstruction caused by large prostate stones. Surgical procedures like open transvesical prostate stone extraction [23], endoscopic extraction [12,22,25], open prostatolithotomy [26] and even radical prostatectomy [27] have been performed to extract these stones.

As mentioned above ,in one study anti-nanobacterial agent was studied in patients with chronic prostatitis and prostate stones and it was shown that prostate stones diminished 50% ultrasonographically [21]. But, yet this is to be clarified by further studies.

6. Summary

In the prostate gland acini, the small round luminal hyaline masses are called corpora amylacea and their calcifications form prostate stones. Suggested mechanism is the intra-prostatic reflux of urine which causes the deposition of hydroxyapatite crystallites in corpora amylacea and mineralization with calcium. Some pathological conditions like alkaptonuria and vitamin D overdose have been reported to cause prostatic calculi. Major calcium components of prostate stone are calcium phosphate or calcium oxalate, along with carbonate-apatite and hydroxyapatite, whereas most prevalent proteins are lactoferrin, myeloperoxidase, and S100 calcium-binding proteins A8 and A9. Being predominantly located in the cephalic portion of the posterior lobe and in the larger ducts and acini of the lateral lobes of the prostate, prostate stones are mostly clinically asymptomatic. When it is symptomatic the symptoms are generally related to lower urinary tract symptoms. Few cases with large prostate stones causing infravesical obstruction and necessitating surgical intervention have been reported. No direct or indirect relationship has been reported between prostate stone and prostate cancer.

7. References

[1] Marx FJ, Karenberg A (2009) History of the term prostate. Prostate. 69:208-213.

[2] Cunha GR, Ricke W, Thomson A, Marker PC, Risbridger G, Hayward SW, Wang YZ, Donjacour AA, Kurita T(2004) Hormonal, cellular, and molecular regulation of normal and neoplastic prostatic development. J Steroid Biochem Mol Biol. 92:221-36.Review.

[3] Cohen RJ, McNeal JE, Redmond SL, Meehan K, Thomas R, Wilce M, Dawkins HJ (2000) Luminal contents of benign and malignant prostatic glands: correspondence to altered secretory mechanisms. Hum Pathol. 31:94-100.

[4] Christian JD, Lamm TC, Morrow JF, Bostwick DG (2005) Corpora amylacea in adenocarcinoma of the prostate: incidence and histology within needle core biopsies. Mod Pathol.18: 36–39.

[5] Moore RA (1936) Morphology of prostatic corpora amylacea. Arch Pathol. 22: 24–40.
[6] Hassler O (1968) Calcification in the prostate gland and adjacent tissues. A combined biophysical and histological study. Path Microbiol. 31: 97–107.
[7] Magura CE, Spector M (1979) Scanning electron microscopy of human prostatic corpora amylacea and corpora calculi, and prostatic calculi. Scan Electron Microsc 3: 713–720.
[8] Köseoğlu H, Aslan G, Sen BH, Tuna B, Yörükoğlu K (2010) Prostatic calculi: silent stones. Actas Urol Esp. 34:555-559.
[9] Young HH (1934) Prostatic calculi. J Urol.32:660–709.
[10] Ramires TC, Ruiz JA, Gomez AZ et al (1980) A crystallographic study of prostatic calculi. J Urol. 124: 840–843.
[11] Izzidien AU (1980) Prostatic calcification in a four year old boy. Arch Dis Child. 55: 963–968.
[12] Strimer RM, Worn LJ (1977) Renal and vesical prostatic calculi associated with ochronosis. Urology.10: 42–34.
[13] Vilches J, Lopez A, De Palacio L, Muñoz C, Gomez J (1982) SEM and X-ray microanalysis of human prostatic calculi. J Urol.127:371-373.
[14] Kodaka T, Hirayama A, Sano T, Debari K, Mayahara M, Nakamura M (2008) Fine structure and mineral components of primary calculi in some human prostates. J Electron Microsc (Tokyo).57:133-141.
[15] Sfanos KS, Wilson BA, De Marzo AM, Isaacs WB (2009) Acute inflammatory proteins constitute the organic matrix of prostatic corpora amylacea and calculi in men with prostate cancer. Proc Natl Acad Sci U S A.106:3443-3448.
[16] Thomas BA, Robert JT (1927) Prostatic calculi. J Urol.18: 470–493.
[17] Lee SE, Ku JH, Park HK, Jeong CK, Kim SH (2003) Prostatic calculi do not influence the level of serum prostate specific antigen in men without clinically detectable prostate cancer or prostatitis. J Urol.170: 745–748.
[18] Kim WB, Doo SW, Yang WJ, Song YS (2011) Influence of prostatic calculi on lower urinary tract symptoms in middle-aged men. Urology.78:447-449.
[19] Park SW, Nam JK, Lee SD, Chung MK (2010) Are prostatic calculi independent predictive factors of lower urinary tract symptoms? Asian J Androl.12:221-226.
[20] Geramoutsos I, Gyftopoulos K, Perimenis P, Thanou V, Liagka D, Siamblis D, Barbalias G (2004) Clinical correlation of prostatic lithiasis with chronic pelvic pain syndromes in young adults. Eur Urol.45:333-337.
[21] Shoskes DA, Thomas KD, Gomez E (2005) Anti-nanobacterial Therapy for men with chronic prostatitis/chronic pelvic pain syndrome and prostatic stones: preliminary experience. J Urol. 73: 474–477.
[22] Hayakawa T, Saito T, Mitsuya H, Kojima M, Hayase Y (2001) [A case of infravesical obstruction caused by prostatic stones as diagnosed by transrectal ultrasonography at voiding]. Hinyokika Kiyo.47.289-292.
[23] Spittel RL (1915) Calculi of the Prostate. Br Med J.21;2(2851):289-91
[24] Kamai T, Toma T, Kano H, Ishıwata D (1999) Urethral obstruction due to protruding prostatic calculi. J Urol.162: 163–164.
[25] Bedir S, Kilciler M, Akay O, Erdemir F, Avci A, Ozgok Y (2005) Endoscopic treatment of multiple prostatic calculi causing urinary retention. Int J Urol.12: 693–695.

[26] Shah SK, Chau MH, Schnepper GD, Lui PD (2007) Open prostatolithotomy for the management of giant prostatic calculi. Urology.70:1008.e9-10.

[27] Virgili G, Forte F, Sansalone S, Attisani F, De Carolis A, Di Stasi SM, Vespasiani G (2004) Radical prostatectomy as unique chance for huge prostatic stones.Arch Ital Urol Androl. 76:171-172.

5

Ureteric Function and Upper Urinary Tract Urodynamics in Patients with Stones in Kidney and Ureter

Mudraya Irina and Khodyreva Lubov
Research Institute of Urology, Russia

1. Introduction

The clinical manifestations of stone disease, its complications and prognosis are closely bound up with the upper urinary tract (UUT) urodynamics. In urological clinical practice, obstruction and peculiarities of pelvicalicael anatomy are usually taken into consideration as the major urodynamic factors in discussions of stone disease pathogenesis (Husmann et al., 1995; Matin & Streem, 2000; Grampsas et al., 2000; Sorensen & Chandhoke, 2002). Less attention is given to the role of functional UUT abnormalities especially in ureteric peristalsis because of designing a method to record human ureteric activity without causing interference is difficult (Shafik, 1996; 1998; Kinn, 1996; Davenport et al., 2007; 2011).

From the viewpoint of UUT physiology, it is known that smooth muscle contractions are essential for urine transport from kidney to the urinary bladder. This process is performed by two major mechanisms: the passive flow driven by hydrostatic pressure, and active one resulted from contractile activity of the smooth muscles in the wall of urinary tract. Both mechanisms are well studied in vivo and in vitro on various animal models under physiological and pathological conditions, and now they are discussed in relation to human urological diseases.

The coordinated muscular contractions propagating along the ureter and providing the active mechanism of urine transport have been generally termed as 'ureteral peristalsis'. Contractions of smooth muscles within UUT are evoked by action potential activity in atypical smooth muscle cells termed interstitial cells of Cajal (ICC)-like cells or pacemaker cells (Hannappel & Golenhofen, 1974; Lang & Klemm, 2005; Pezzone, et al., 2003; McHale et al., 2006; Hashitani et al., 2009; Lee et al., 2011). The role of the ICC-like system in the urinary tract is discussed in relation to variety of severe congenital and/or acquired urological diseases, such as hydroureter and megaloureter (McHale et al., 2006). Whether these atypical pacemaker activities within ureter can disorganize UUT peristalsis has not been elucidated for the stone disease. However, it was demonstrated that excitation of latent pacemakers by noxious/irritant stimuli occurring during a passage of a stone or a bacterial infection can generate the antiperistaltic contractile waves producing urine reflux toward the kidney (Santicioli & Maggi, 1998). Moreover, in a divided ureter, the normal antegrade electrical activity can be replaced by retrograde contractions occurring in different UUT parts independently (Tindall, 1972). Cellular and molecular processes directing normal ureter development as well as disease mechanisms leading to obstructive uropathies are still unknown (Airik, et al., 2010). Coordinating proximal-to-distal peristalsis of the upper urinary tract is commonly defective in congenital diseases (Hurtado, et al., 2010). However, in clinical trials, functional disturbances in UUT are little examined, and there are only limited data on the role of ureteral peristalsis in the course of stone disease (Davenport et al., 2006, 2011).

Under the resting conditions, regular UUT electrical and contractile function is characteristic of normal peristaltic urine transport. The action potentials spreading to the membrane of ureteral smooth muscle cells induce their contractions employing the mechanisms common for other smooth muscles. The rhythmic contractions of ureter are driven by propagating membrane depolarization. Myogenic and neurogenic nature of muscle contraction is still discussed on the basis of calcium and Rho-kinase cellular contractility mechanisms and peculiarities of UUT innervation (Kobayashi 1965; Notley, 1971; Santicioli & Maggi, 1998; Levent & Buyukafsar, 2004; Weiss et al., 2006; Hurtado, et al., 2010; Grisk, et al., 2010).

Enhancement in urine production results in stretching the ureter and increasing the volume of urinary bolus. The increasing urinary flow is accompanied with growing rate of peristaltic contractions till the ureter takes the shape of an open duct (Constantinou, 1974; Constantinou & Yamaguchi, 1981; Harada et al., 1984; Kim et al., 2002). In such cases, urine passage is passive, which does not use peristaltic movement of ureteric wall, so urine is driven entirely by hydrostatic pressure gradient from the areas of high pressure to those of low pressure.

The role of intraluminal pressure in the UUT was thoroughly discussed for experimental physiological and pathological conditions, as well as for clinical settings (Davis, 1954). It was shown that pressure developed by peristaltic wave is responsible for the unidirectional transport of urinary bolus being therefore a kind of "active" antireflux mechanism. Contractile function of proximal and distal ureteral segments and the influence of baseline ureteral distending pressure upon ureteral luminal pressure generation are discussed with respect to ureteral function during urinary outflow obstruction (Rasidovic et al., 2010). Moreover, there are data indicating peristaltic pressure as a vital requirement for the complex process of urine secretion, conduction, storage, and expulsion from the body. Peristaltic contractions of the pelvic wall were proved to be an effective mechanism that concentrates urine in the renal papilla (Dwyer & Schmidt-Nielsen, 2003). At present, the pressure measurements have been used to study medication effects on ureteral peristalsis (Davenport et al., 2006; Pick et al., 2011) or they are fulfilled in order to protect kidney from harmful pressure increase during ureteroscopy (Jung et al., 2006; Page et al., 2011; Jung & Osther, 2011). Despite essential role of this urodynamic phenomenon for renal function, the dynamic changes in the renal pelvis pressure during stone disease course were little studied.

The above shortly described physiological mechanisms of ureter functioning can be helpful to explain the urodynamic disorders in patients with stone disease. Objective information on ureteral function status in each patient, the knowledge on urodynamic transporting mechanism, whether it happens by passive hydrodynamic flow or by active peristalsis, can be useful to prognosticate and avoid the possible complications such as urine stagnation and refluxes.

2. Methods of the UUT urodynamic functional diagnostics

In clinical practice, visualization methods are commonly used to assess urodynamic disorders. They are based on ultrasound, X-ray, isotopic, and magnetic resonance examinations yielding information on UUT size and structure, and on stone or stricture location (Kinn, 1996). The qualitative data on ureteral function given by visualization techniques is UUT dilation, and an indication on peristaltic frequency (Kim et al., 2008).

In experimental studies, more functional parameters are harvested by physiological methods, but these possibilities are seldom used in clinical setting. The physiological measurements include electromyography, as well as impedance and intraluminal pressure measurements along a ureter.

Electromyographic studies have established the characteristics of ureteric excitation (Shafik, 1996; Roshani et al., 2000). The impedance measurements are based on field gradient principle for quantification of cross sectional area of ureteral urine bolus (Harada et al., 1984), or as a function of ureteric motor activity (Roshani et al., 1999 2000; Kinn, & Lykkeskov-Andersen, 2002).

Electromyography together with impedance method based on cross sectional area of urine bolus measurement was reported to be carried out in laboratory and clinical experiments (Harada et al., 1984). The authors used the probe consisted of ureteral catheter with 4 ring impedance electrodes and a bipolar ring ureteromyographic electrode. As urine bolus passed through the impedance electrodes, the value of impedance represented the cross sectional area of the urine bolus.

As a function of ureteric motor activity, the impedance measured between thin copper electrodes placed on a catheter in two sites 10 cm apart enabled to analyze frequency, direction, and velocity of peristaltic waves (Kinn, & Lykkeskov-Andersen, 2002). With a single catheter recording EMG, impedance, and the pressure changes, the characteristics of mechanical activity during ureteral peristalsis, propagation velocity of the peristaltic wave through ureter, and urine bolus transport were quantified (Roshani et al., 1999).

For simultaneous study of electrical and mechanical parameters of ureteral peristalsis in pigs, electrical potentials from ureter were lead with bipolar steel-wire electromyography electrodes delivered laparoscopically, and the mechanical movements were monitored by giant magneto resistive sensors mounted on custom-made aluminium strips (Venkatesh et al., 2005; Page et al., 2011).

Peristaltic frequency, conduction velocity, and intraureteral pressure was assessed in an animal model and in six patients who had undergone ureteroscopy with the commercial ureteral pressure transducer catheter (Young et al., 2007). It was demonstrated that instrumented human ureter displayed a variable response related to previous physical or pharmacologic effects.

Ureteric peristalsis characterized with contraction frequency, pressure and velocity measurements was recorded in eighteen patients with the help of ureteric pressure transducer catheter (Davenport et al., 2007). The authors concluded that despite various limitations intrinsic to ureteric catheters, these measurements provide some useful information when used to record the response to an intervention in the same patient.

In our experimental study we simultaneously recorded electromyogram, electromagnetically measured urine flow rate, intraluminal pressure, and impedance via special probes consecutively applied to the same ureter in dog (Fig.1). This record illustrates physiological events in the ureter obtained by direct measurements. The electromyogram spikes precede the peaks of flow wave that initiates pressure rise and corresponds well in time to impedance oscillations. The ureteric impedance decreases maximally during the passage of the urine bolus associated with maximal increase in the flow volume curve.

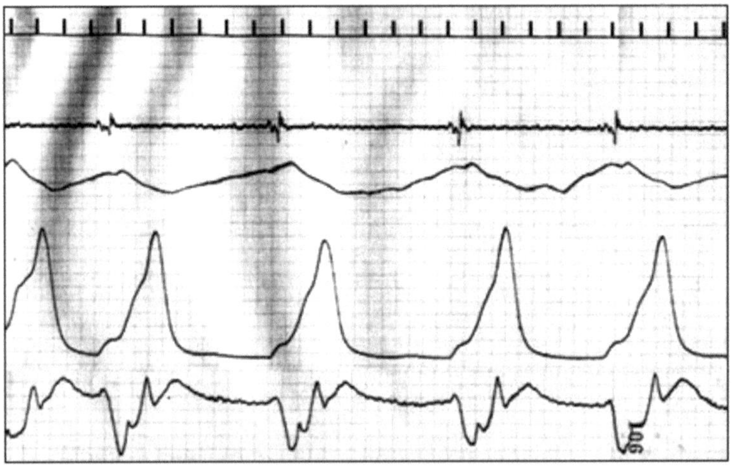

Fig. 1. An example of simultaneous ureteric peristalsis registration in a healthy anesthetized dog. Channels (top-down): time controller (1 sec); electroureterogram (mV); urine flow rate (ml/min); pressure (cm H_2O); impedance ureterogram (Ohm)

Thus, the routine recording of ureteric excitation can be supplemented with the data on mechanical activity during ureteral peristalsis assessed with impedance and pressure measurements. Anyway, very little data are available on ureteral peristalsis in the clinical settings, which actualizes functional diagnostic of urodynamic conditions in patients with stones in UUT.

In our further work, multichannel ureter impedance recordings were used to study ureteral function under normal and pathological conditions in dog experiments, and also in clinical examinations of urological patients with stone disease, hydro- and ureterohydronephrosis (Mudraya et al., 2001; 2007; 2011).

The multichannel impedance ureterography (MIUG) method is carried out using a 8F probe inserted into a ureter of a patient endoscopically. The measuring probe is equipped with 9 consecutively incorporated separate electrodes. The current (2 mA and 32 kHz frequency) is driven to extreme (the 1st and the 9th) electrodes of the probe while the interim electrodes served for impedance measurements. The potential differences from the consecutive pairs of measuring electrodes (2-3; 3-4; 4-5; 5-6; 6-7; 7-8) permit to obtain the impedance waveform of the adjacent parts of the ureter during its activity. The impedance converter "RPKA2-01" ("Medass", Russia) and special software (MCDP32) provides simultaneous 6-channel monitoring of the instantaneous impedances within consecutive ureter segments.

The assessment of the function of a ureter is fulfilled automatically and processed according to the following parameters at impedance ureterogram as Fig. 2 shows. The peristalsis amplitude (A) is the maximal deflection of impedance during urine bolus passage and contraction of ureter. The ureteral wall tone (T) is an inverse value of impedance deflection taking place immediately to rhythmic breath activity. The peristalsis rate (f) is calculated from time period between consecutive contractions. The duration of a contractile wave (D) is a distance between the start and the end point of ureteral contraction corresponding to impedance curve deflection from isoelectric line. Calculation of conduction velocity was made using a single contraction recorded by six electrode pairs on the probe - the velocity of contractile wave (or urine bolus propagation V) is the product of division of the constant distance between the first and the last pair of potential electrodes (75 mm) and the time needed for propagation of the wave along this distance. In addition to quantitative parameters of ureteric function, the multichannel impedance monitoring made it possible to evaluate the qualitative characteristics of UUT peristalsis. These parameters include the shape and direction of the peristaltic wave propelling (antegrade, retrograde, cystoid, chaotic), and their rhythmicity. The normal (antegrade) peristaltic wave usually appears in the upper regions and spreads down the ureter (Fig.3, a). The retrograde (reflux) contractile wave propagates in the opposite direction that can be reliably monitored (c). Cystoid contractions recorded with MIUG represent simultaneous contractions in ureteral region 7.5 cm in length (ureteral cystoid located across the probe), which is equal to the distance between the 1st and the last 6th pair of registering electrodes on the probe (b, d).

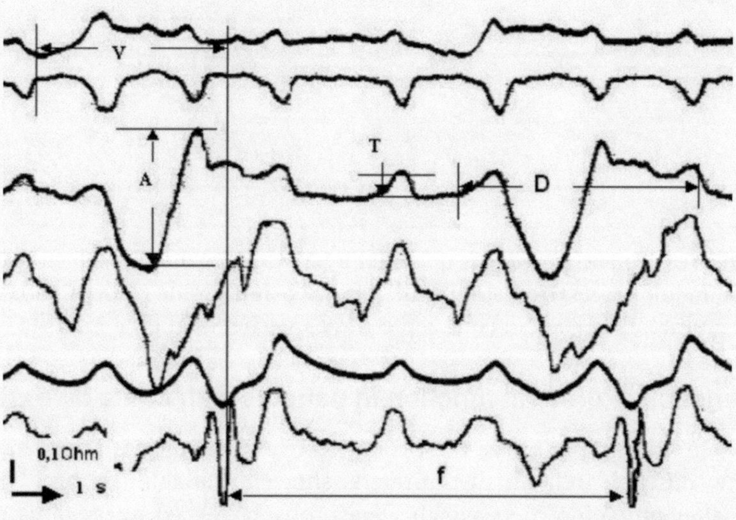

Fig. 2. Example of MIUG with ureteral peristalsis parameters. A- peristalsis amplitude; T- ureteral wall tone; D- duration of a contractile wave; f- time period between consecutive contractions; V- velocity of contractile wave

Here our experience is described on MIUG and intrapelvic pressure measurements performed within the routine of complex urodynamic examination of the patients with stone disease. On the whole, 250 patients with various urolithiasis clinical histories were randomly involved and examined in different patients groups composed according to duration and severity of stone obstruction, inflammatory complications, and some treatment procedures. The status of UUT urodynamics was assessed with standard ultrasonic and X-ray examinations. MIUG method has been employed in patients during diagnostic ureteroscopy (URS), lithotripsy procedures and ureteral stent exchanging. Electromanometric pressure measurements were fulfilled in patients who had clinical indication to nephrostomy. The renal pelvic pressure (RPP) measurements have been performed via nephrostomy tube in the course of obstructive stone disease management and inflammatory complication medical or operative treatment.

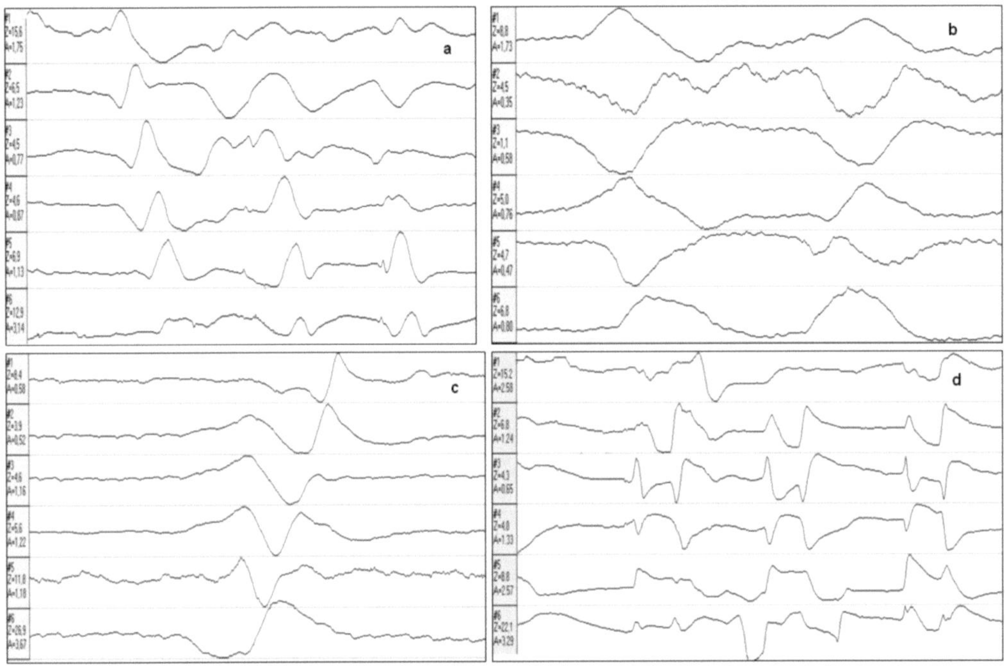

Fig. 3. Examples of ureteral peristalsis obtained by MIUG in patients with stone disease. a- antegrade contractile waves; b- cystoid contractions; c- retrograde (reflux) peristaltic wave; d- deformed multitoothed cystoid contractile waves; each record time is 20 sec

3. Characteristics of ureteral function in patients with stone disease.

Abnormalities in ureteral peristalsis were common in all patients with urolithiasis although their severity differed individually. Ureters showed variable patterns of peristalsis immediately after probe insertion, which were probably related to previous physiological and pathological conditions.

On the whole, the patients with stones in UUT were characterized with decreased amplitude of ureteric peristalsis, increased ureteral wall tone, and larger peristalsis rate as compared to the normal ureters (Table 1). The data were obtained in 43 patients with UUT stones before lithotripsy session (of them 7 patients with solitary kidney) and 3 patients with normal ureters during diagnostic URS.

Parameters	Ureteral segment		
	proximal	middle	distal
Patients with both kidneys			
Peristalsis amplitude (Ohm)	0.70±0.08	0.61±0.15	0.61±0.13
Ureteral wall tone (Ohm^{-1})	5.5±0.9	4.5±1.4	5.8±1.3
Peristalsis frequency (min^{-1})	3.2±0.8	3.1±0.6	3.8±0.9
Solitary-kidney patients			
Peristalsis amplitude (Ohm)	1.12±0.25	1.18±0.26	1.11±0.23
Ureteral wall tone (Ohm^{-1})	4.2±0.5	2.5±0.4	4.7±2.5
Peristalsis frequency (min^{-1})	4.6±1.4	6.5±1.4	4.4±1.8
Patients without stone in the UUT			
Peristalsis amplitude (Ohm)			2.1±0.9
Ureteral wall tone (Ohm^{-1})			2.2±1.4
Peristalsis frequency (min^{-1})			2.0±0.7

Table 1. Parameters of ureteral peristalsis in patients with stones in UUT and patients with normal ureters

Three patients with normal ureters were subjected to diagnostic URS for roentgen-negative stones. Of them, two patients had unilateral UUT stones, and one patient had a benign prostate hyperplasia. No stones or urodynamic disorders were revealed in the examined ureters of these patients. All of them demonstrated the examples of rhythmic antegrade peristalsis in distal ureteral cystoid. In the normal ureter, urine is propelled antegradely towards the bladder, while the contractions spread downstream along the ureter.

Among the patients with stone disease, there were those whose ureters demonstrated pronounced activity with differently directed contractile waves in the ureter (Fig.4, a). In addition, there were patients with aberrant chaotic peristalsis (Fig. 4, b). These parameters were characteristic of each patient's ureteral peristalsis and in average did not significantly differ in the upper, middle, or distal cystoid of the ureter. In the patients who had solitary kidney, the ureteral function differed from that in the patients with both kidneys. In the case of solitary kidney, enhanced peristalsis amplitude and higher rate of contractile activity attest to hyperfunction of the ureter (Table 1).

According to the mean values of peristalsis amplitude and ureteral wall tone, 33 patients with stone disease were divided into four groups (Table 2). It is supposed the high amplitude rhythmic contractions and the low wall tone are characteristic of the normal ureteral function (Table 2, group I). Such peristalsis was observed only in 23% patients examined with MIUG, whose ureters looked like the normal ones. However, the most often characteristic of the ureteral function in examined patients with stones in UUT was combination of the low amplitude of contractions with enhanced ureteral wall tone indicating severe dysfunction in ureteric peristalsis (Table 2, group IV). Such peculiarities in ureter performance were observed in 42% patients. These quantitative characteristics are corroborated by observations on the increasing number of the patients with peristaltic arrhythmia, contractile wave deformity (e.g. the appearance of the multitoothed contractions) and peristaltic disturbances manifested by retrograde and cystoid waves.

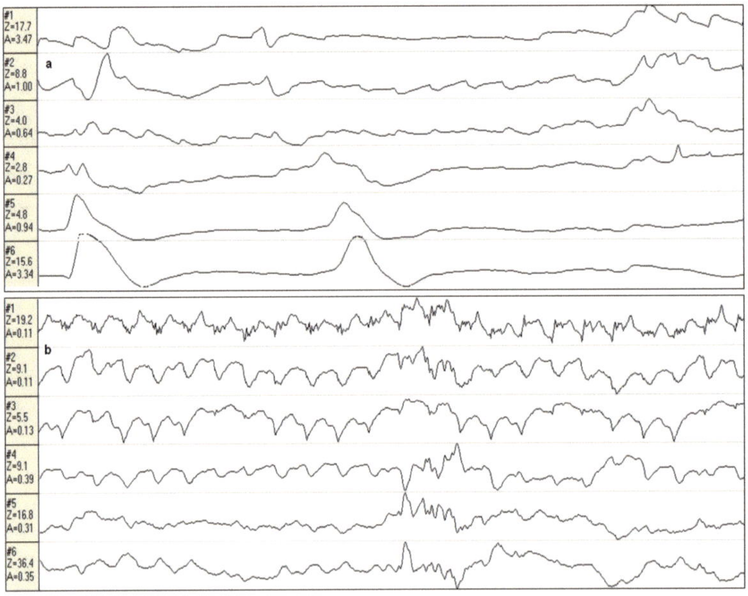

Fig. 4. Examples of ureteral peristalsis obtained by MIUG in patients with a- strong contractile activity in the ureter, and b,- with aberrant peristalsis; each record time is 20 sec

Patient groups	I	II	III	IV
Peristalsis amplitude (Ohm)	1.8±0.4	1.3±0.2	0.5±0.1	0.3±0.03
Ureteral wall tone (Ohm^{-1})	2.2±0.1	7.9±1.8	2.9±0.2	13.2±2.1
Peristalsis frequency per minute	2.6±0.2	2.2±0.6	3.3±0.3	3.0±0.2
Qualitative peristalsis characteristics (manifestation percentage)				
Arrhythmia	52±6	30±5	86±8	84±7
Deformed contractions	51±3	50±3	71±6	84±5
Antegrade waves	100	68±4	19±3	34±5
Retrograde waves	50±4	50±5	73±6	87±7
Cystoid contractions	16±3	43±5	91±9	86±8

Table 2. Parameters of ureteral peristalsis in patients with stone disease according to MIUG data

Thus, the antegrade propagation of peristaltic waves along the ureter was characteristic of the normal ureteral peristalsis. It is reliable to show that in normal ureter, peristaltic wave travels from proximal to distal cystoid, i.e. antegradely. This antegrade peristalsis ensures urine transport from renal pelvis towards the bladder and serves to protect renal parenchyma, while the backflow of urine generated by retrograde contractile waves can induce back pressure and urine refluxes that are dangerous for kidney (Davis, 1954; Dwyer & Schmidt-Nielsen, 2003; Mudraya & Khodyreva, 2011). The cystoid contractions are supposed to represent simultaneous motion in ureteral cystoid that is likely referred to diuretic mode of urine transport through opened and dilated ureter. The deformed multitoothed contractions and peristalsis arrhythmia can be the features of ureteral wall irritation and repeated excitations of smooth muscle cells. These data corroborate the opinion that irritation and stretch stimulation of the ureter by a stone may result in large uncoordinated peristalsis (Rose & Gillenwater, 1973; Davenport et al., 2006).

Among the examined patients, we couldn't find the differences in ureteral function depending on the patients' age and gender. However, the urolithiasis history was essential for appearance of ureteral function. The special features of peristalsis were observed in patients with renal colic, primordial, or permanent stones. They will be discussed further. In general, there was a tendency to smaller ureteral peristalsis amplitude (0.51±0.16 Ohm) and higher (by 23%) ureteral wall tone in the patients suffering from stone disease for a long time, compared to the patients having stones for only short periods (1.16±0.34 Ohm). The cystoid and retrograde contractions were prevailing among other kinds of peristaltic activity in the ureters of patients with long-term stone disease history, and the peristalsis rate was slower by 48% in them than in the patients who had stones for several months only (Fig. 5).

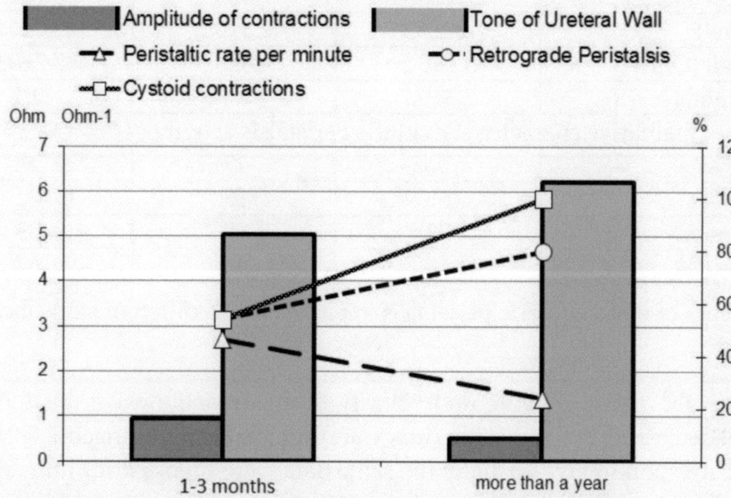

Fig. 5. General dynamics of ureter functional parameters in relation to duration of stone disease

4. Peculiarities of the ureteral function in patients with various stone position in UUT

Analysis of ureteral function has been performed for thirty patients with renal (8) and ureteral (22) stones in UUT. Of 8 patients with renal stones, 7 patients had unilateral and 1 had bilateral calculi. Of 22 patients with ureteral stones, 12 had urolith in the proximal ureter, while other had it in distal ureter (one patient had bilateral stones). In these patients, the diagnostic probe has been introduced into the distal ureteral cystoid, and peristalsis in the distal part of ureter was evaluated by MIUG.

Despite the fact that ureteral function parameters differed to a great extent among the patients, the peculiar features were observed in patients with various stone position in UUT (table 3). The average data show that patients with distal stones in UUT were characterized with decreased amplitude of ureteric peristalsis and increased ureteral wall tone compared to the patients with kidney and proximal ureteral stones. Thus, peristalsis was mostly seriously disturbed and destroyed in the region of stone location. The weak irregular contractions were typical for the patients with distal ureteral stones (67%). Evident cystoid and retrograde contractions as well as poor chaotic peristalsis were typical for the patients with proximal ureteral stones. The peristalsis amplitude in these patients was higher than that in patients with distal stones but lower than that in patients with renal stones. Most patients with renal stones (82%) demonstrated active ureteral peristalsis: the contractile waves of antegrade as well as retrograde direction were observed along with ureteral cystoid contractions. The mean peristalsis amplitude was the highest in them compared to others, while the tone was the lowest than in patients with other stone location.

Parameters	Renal stones	Upper ureter stones	Distal ureter stones
Peristalsis amplitude (Ohm)	1.08±0.12	0.63±0.08	0.45±0.04
Duration of a contraction (s)	7.1±0.4	7.6±0.2	8.1±1.1
Peristalsis rate (min^{-1})	2.9±0.1	2.8±0.2	2.7±0.8
Tone of ureteral wall (Ohm^{-1})	4.2±0.5	4.8±0.3	7.2±0.9
Velocity of contraction (cm/s)	2.3±0.7	2.9	2.1
Qualitative characteristics of the peristalsis activity			
Antegrade waves (%)	56	17	22
Retrograde waves (%)	66	83	22
Cystoid contractions (%)	33	67	33
Aberrant peristalsis (%)	18	40	67

Table 3. Characteristics of distal ureteric peristalsis in patients with different stone location in UUT

The average data on the peristalsis rate and velocity of a contractile wave obtained with MIUG in normal patients and in those with kidney and ureteral stones ranged 2.0-2.9 min^{-1} and 1.3–2.9 cm/s, correspondingly. Virtually the same data were reported for human ureter obtained by intraluminal ureteric pressure measurements: the peristalsis rate and conduction velocity respectively ranged 0–4.1 min^{-1} and 1.5–2.6 cm/s (Davenport et al., 2007). Visualization technique yielded only the data for peristaltic rate 3.5 min^{-1} in normal ureters, while the abnormal ureters were characterized with decreased or absent peristalsis (Kim et al., 2008).

Moreover, the results obtained with MIUG method showed that the following three parameters differed in the ureters with stones despite of their position from the ureters with no stones. The velocity of contraction tended to be greater by 64-125% in ureters with stone compared to the normal ureters (1.3±0.3 cm/s). In such ureters, the peristalsis rate was faster by 35-81% than the normal rate of 2.0±0.7 min^{-1}, while the contractile wave duration was shorter by 13-28% (compared to the normal value of 9.9±0.8 s). Such results may reflect the specificity of ureteral peristalsis in patients with uroliths in UUT. Probably, the stone-induced irritations trigger rapid and simultaneous (cystoid) contractions of the ureter. The pronounced organic changes in ureteral wall due to fibrotic processes are usually characterized by aberrant peristalsis in the region of stone location. In the case of proximal stones in UUT, the peristalsis disturbances and strong contractile activity in distal ureter can be explained by reflex irritation of ureteral wall with a stone. Diagrams 1-4 (Fig. 6) well demonstrate differences in the parameters of ureteral peristalsis depending on stone position in UUT assessed by MIUG method.

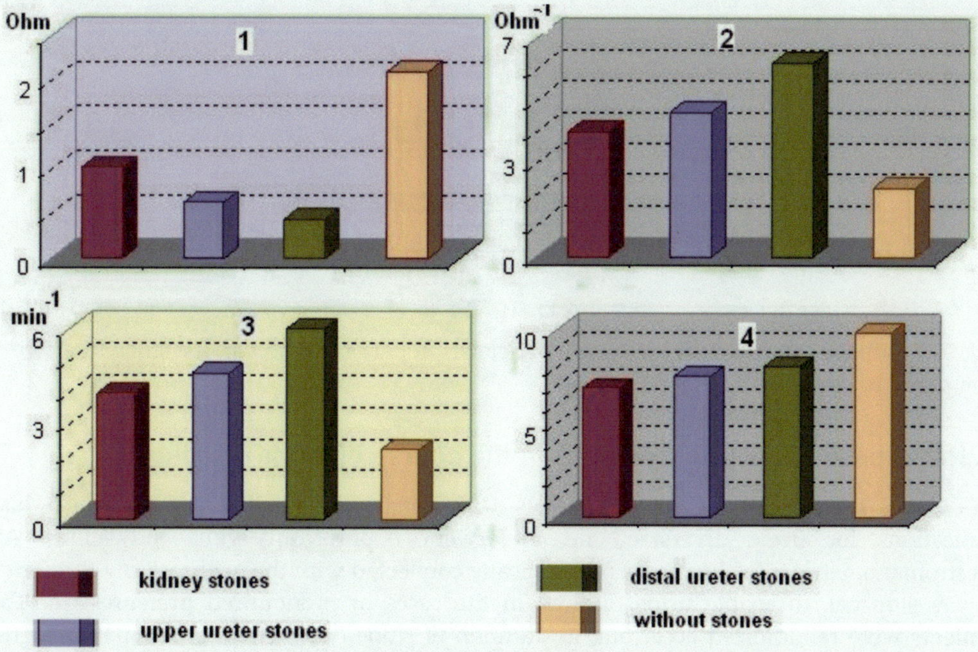

Fig. 6. Quantitative parameters of ureteric peristalsis in patients with various stone location compared to controls. 1- peristalsis amplitude; 2- ureteral wall tone; 3- peristalsis rate; 4- contractile wave duration

Thus, special features of ureteral peristalsis were observed in the patients with various stone position in UUT. Peristalsis amplitude was weaker, ureteral wall tone was higher, and contractile waves were faster and shorter in the ureters of patients with stones in the upper urinary tract as compared to the control group.

Figure 7 demonstrates that patients with the combination of differently directed contractile waves (antegrade, retrograde, cystoid) were numerous in a group with the renal stones. The antegrade contractile waves were observed in 50% patients with renal stones, and only in 9-12% patients with stones in ureter. The cystoid contractions were characteristic to all patients with uroliths in UUT (50-63%). The retrograde contractile waves in ureter were often observed in patients with the renal (67%) and proximal ureteral stones (54%), while the aberrant peristalsis was often recorded in patients with the ureteral stones (proximal - distal, 45-69%), in contrast to patients with the renal stones (10%).

The underlying mechanisms of urodynamic disorders seem to be different in patients with different stone position. Our data suggest that proximal UUT stones can disturb ureteral function producing vigorous uncoordinated contractions. On the contrary, the stones disposed in distal ureter which disturb its peristalsis can affect renal pelvic urodynamics, induce elevation in RPP, and/or dilation of the pelvicaliceal system.

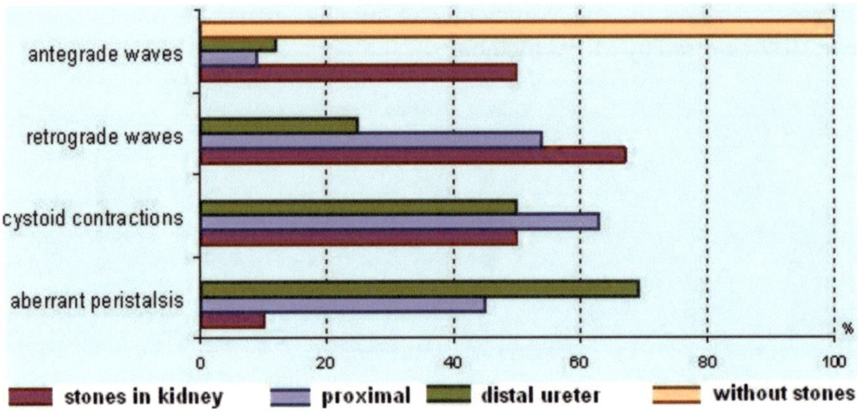

Fig. 7. Qualitative parameters of ureteric peristalsis in patients with various stone location compared to controls

5. Renal pelvis pressure dynamics in the course of stone disease

RPP have been measured in 73 patients with renal and ureteral stones, which had indications for urine diversion and underwent nephrostomy tube indwelling. An electromanometric transducer was hydraulically connected with the nephrostomy through a 3-way stopcock to enable urine outflow in the cases of pronounced pressure rise. The patients were randomized according to duration of stone obstruction, inflammation signs, the treatment history, and the level of obstruction.

Despite individual changes in the mean RPP in patients with UUT stones, analysis revealed different role of obstruction and inflammation in pressure elevation (Fig.8). The highest baseline pressure values in renal pelvis were recorded in the patients, who had stone obstruction accompanied with inflammation within up to 4-day period (25.0±1.6 cm H_2O) and 5-10-day period (28.7±2.6 cm H_2O). In the patients with ureters obstructed for 1-4 days that had no signs of inflammation, RPP was only moderately elevated (14.7±2.9 cm H_2O).

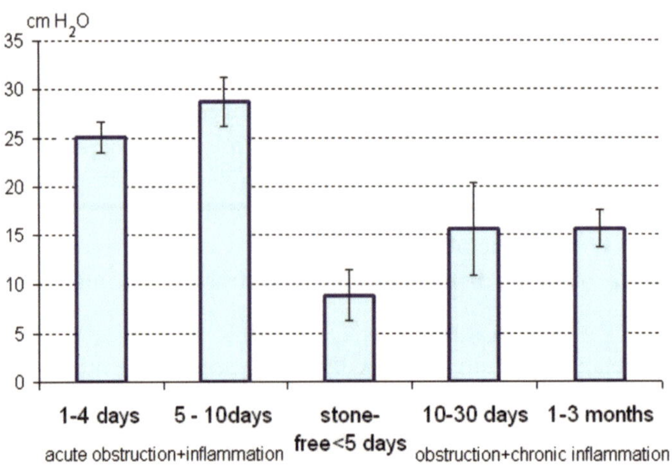

Fig. 8. Mean baseline RPP in stone disease patients in the course of treatment

In the unobstructed patients, in case of the short-term obstruction resolving, RPP quickly gave a reasonable fit to a normal sense (3.6±1.4 cm H_2O). It is accepted that the normal baseline RPP values make up 10 cm H_2O measured in voluntaries (Shafic, 1998).

Thus, the results evidence that the main reasons of RPP rise in the patients with stones in UUT is obstruction and inflammation timing. The data on especially high RPP values registered on days 5-10 of acute inflammatory complication of obstruction, but not within the first 4 days, probably indicate significance of simultaneous rise in renal interstitial pressure and the development of inflammation progression, that is, the pressure in the intercellular spaces of the kidney (Davis, 1954). Smaller pressure variations produced by peristalsis or transmitted respiratory activity in renal pelvis during acute inflammation seems to corroborate this view. According to our results, the baseline RPP was higher (26.4±1.5 cm H_2O) in the acute period of inflammation and obstruction (up to 10 day-period) than during chronic inflammation (15.6±1.9 cm H_2O), while the mean delta pressure was much lesser in them (1.9±0.2 vs 4.8±0.3 cm H_2O), respectively. As this urodynamic parameter changes individually within a short or a long-term course of the stone disease, RPP can be considered as a reliable index of inflammation resolving and obstruction rescuing in patients, and therefore it can be used to predict future renal status.

The value of RPP depended on the level of obstruction being higher than 10 cm H2O in the most of patients (90%) with distally located stones in UUT, and only in 59% patients with renal and proximal ureteral stones. In the 1-month period of obstruction and inflammation, the mean RPP was higher in the patients with distally obstructed ureters than in those patients that had ureters with proximally located concrements (21.8±0.8 vs 12.4±1.2 cm H_2O). However, during the later period of stone obstruction and chronic inflammation (1-3 months), RPP was quite similar in the case of distal as well as proximal stones (16.2±0.7 vs 16.9±0.8 cm H_2O).

RPP is an integral complex urodynamic parameter reflecting urine inflow (the quantity excreting by a kidney), elastic properties of the surrounding UUT wall, and the resistance to urine outflow depending on ureter capability and function. Eleven patients with partial obstruction and chronic inflammation who had nephrostomy were assessed by RPP measurements and following MIUG examination during URS. In them, special associations were noted between urodynamic disorders manifested by RPP elevation and ureteric peristalsis (Table. 4). Among patients with moderately increased RPP, 45% persons demonstrated weak ureteral contractions and pronounced ureteral wall tone. However, ureteric function was characterized by strong uncoordinated contractions and low ureteral wall tone in 36% patients.

RPP (cm H_2O)		Characteristics of Ureteral Contractile Activity			Ureteral wall tone (Ohm^{-1})
Baseline	Peristaltic	Amplitude (Ohm)	Duration (sec)	Frequency (min^{-1})	
14.0±2.5	17.2±2.4	1.04±0.06	7.08±0.28	3.2±0.2	3.4±0.2
16.4±1.3	23.1±3.4	0.29±0.03	7.68±0.61	3.1±0.6	6.8±0.7

Table 4. Characteristics of UUT urodynamics with respect to contractile function of distal ureter in patients with moderately elevated RPP

Thus, the mechanism underlying pressure elevation in renal pelvis varies with respect to ureteral function characterized by peristalsis amplitude and ureteral wall tone. Moreover, it seems to be different in the cases of renal and ureteral stone location. In the group with renal stones, RPP was pronouncedly elevated (>20 cm H_2O) in those patients that demonstrated persistent retrograde and cystoid waves, but it did not exceed 10 cm H_2O in the patients whose ureter demonstrated antegrade contractions. In the group with ureteral stones, an elevated RPP (>10 cm H_2O) was observed in the patients with weak chaotic peristalsis and enhanced ureteral wall tone. So, evident retrograde and cystoid peristaltic waves are supposed to provoke refluxes and urine stagnation contributing to pressure elevation similar to what takes place in patients with renal stones. Also, an aberrant peristalsis and increased ureteral wall tone correlated with elevated RPP and therefore induce urine stagnation as in the patients with ureteral stones.

Some important observations were made in the patients with residual stone fragments remaining in UUT for more than 1 month accompanied by chronic inflammation. Despite persistent adequate renal drainage per nephrostomy tube, RPP was moderately increased in these patients. Moreover, the patients that had lithotripsy procedures in anamnesis demonstrated even higher mean RPP (18.2±1.3, range 3.0 - 26.4 cm H_2O) compared to the patients with no previous lithotripsy procedures (15.6±1.9, range 2 - 18.8 cm H_2O). Moreover, the unobstructed patients without stones in UUT that have been examined before nephrostomy removal, demonstrated higher mean RPP if they had undergone operative treatment (18.9±2.6, range 9.0 - 24.0 cm H_2O) compared with the patients that had not been subjected to such treatment (13.3±1.2, range 9.0 - 20.0 cm H_2O). These results evidence that the operative treatment can affect RPP value.

Acute effects of lithotripsy procedures have been shown to manifest with rapid and short (several seconds) elevations in RPP up to 80 cm H_2O during some phases of the contact lithotripsy, and slow (several minutes) RPP elevations up to 34 cm H_2O were observed during ESWL sessions (Mudraya & Khodyreva 2011). We suppose those acute RPP elevations during lithotripsy sessions could be one of the mechanisms underlying moderate and stable renal pelvis hypertension. The importance to prevent chronically increased intrapelvic pressure is of concern (Davis, 1954). Nowadays, the procedures and medication to avoid sharp pressure rise during URS treatment are developing (Page et al., 2011; Jung & Osther 2011).

6. Efficacy of lithotripsy session in dependence on ureteral function and disorders in urodynamics

The results of extracorporeal shockwave lithotripsy (ESWL) procedure were evaluated in 36 patients according to stone-free rate, steinstrasse formation or residual stones in UUT with respect to stone disease history, and the ureteral functional parameters prior to this ESWL session.

As fig.9 shows, the best treatment results were achieved in the patients with colic demonstrating 60% stone-free rate, while the rate of residual stone formation was the highest in the patients who had stones in UUT for more than a month and ESWL sessions in anamnesis. Steinstrasse was often observed in patients who had surgery for stones (51%). The ureteral function in patients with short (1-4 days) period of stone disease was characterized with widely different contractile activity in ureteral parts before urgent ESWL.

The peristalsis amplitude was the highest (0.76±0.26 Ohm) in the proximal ureter, while ureteral wall tone was especially elevated in the distal region of ureter (8.68±1.41 Ohm^{-1}). Arrhythmic (67%), retrograde (80%), and cystoid contractions (100%) were dominant over the antegrade peristaltic waves in the upper, middle, and distal ureteral segments, respectively.

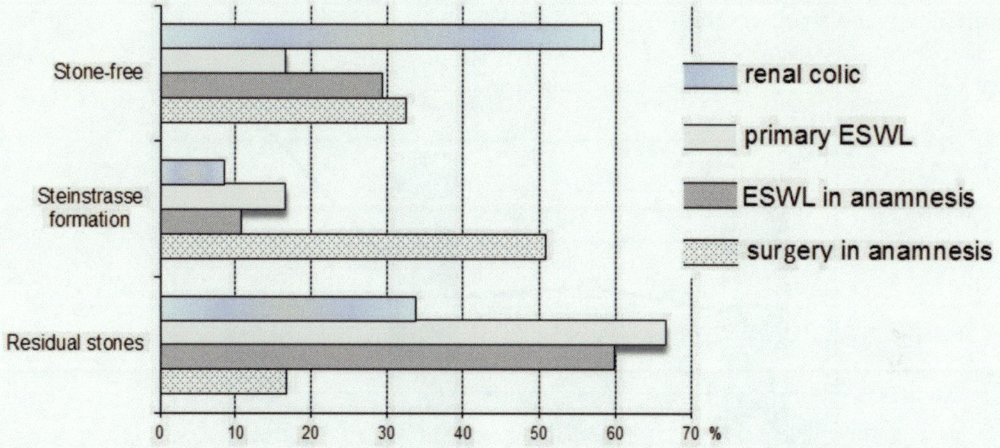

Fig. 9. Results of ESWL session with respect to stone disease history

Despite these peristalsis disorders, the most patients with colic episodes achieved successful stone removal after a single ESWL session. Long-term observation showed that these patients remained stone-free within 3-year follow up period. Only one (of seven) patient had inflammatory complications during the nearest postoperative period followed by nephrostomy. In this patient, high ureteral wall tone and vigorous retrograde contractions in the distal ureter were characteristic for ureteral peristalsis recorded by MIUG before ESWL session, and RPP recordings performed via nephrostomy tube showed rhythmic pressure elevations up to 30 cm H_2O evidently related to the retrograde ureteral contractions.

On the whole, the results evidence that the peristaltic derangement observed during the short-term period of urolothiasis might be reversible after emergent stone-obstruction removal. Thus, one can speculate that the patients with a short-term history of stone disease have safe ureteral smooth muscle wall function. In these patients, the peristalsis disorders observed prior to ESWL originate mainly from the reflex provoked by a stone not from organic changes in ureteral wall. Consequently, ability of ureter to propel urine properly can be quickly restored after restoration of its lumen patency.

The functional urodynamic disorders were pronouncedly aggravating during elongation of stones in UUT, and they changed individually in the course of treatment. Severe disorders in the ureteral peristalsis can be the complicating factor.

Taking into consideration the peculiarities of ureteral function (Fig.10), the high rate of steinstrasse formation can be explained by the weakest peristalsis amplitude and the highest ureteral wall tone in patients with surgery in anamnesis, compared to other patient groups. On the contrary, the high rate of residual stone formation in the patients having stones in UUT for more than a month and subjected to ESWL can be explained by the strong peristalsis amplitude (69%) and frequent incidence of retrograde peristaltic waves (36%). In the patients without ESWL in anamnesis, the retrograde contractions were persistent only in 20% persons, while the rest 80% patients demonstrated weak peristaltic activity. Their peristalsis assumed cystoid (42%) character. In these patients, the high rate of residual stone formation was also observed.

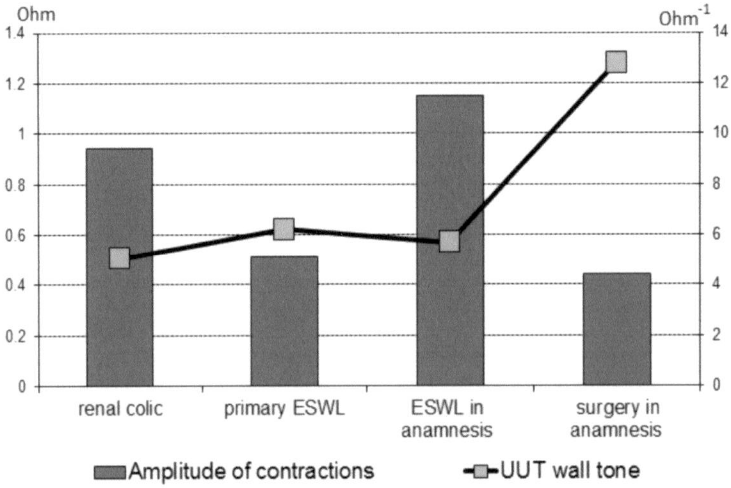

Fig. 10. Parameters of ureteral function obtained with MIUG immediately before ESWL session in patients with different stone disease history

The data on the greater ureteric peristalsis amplitude in patients with lithotripsy in anamnesis in comparison with the primary patients receiving only medication well agree with previously demonstrated higher values of RPP in the patient groups with nephrostomy. The primary patients who had no lithotripsy procedures in anamnesis were characterized with smaller mean RPP, and lesser peristalsis amplitude in ureters, as compared to the patients with ESWL in anamnesis.

Acute effect of another lithotripsy procedure on the parameters of ureteric function was evaluated in 12 patients who underwent contact lithotripsy (CLT). Of them, one patient was assessed by MIUG immediately during CLT session, 6 patients were examined by MIUG and RPP measurements before CLT, and 5 patients were examined after CLT (fig. 11).

In one patient examined immediately during CLT, peristalsis amplitude decreased by 45-50%, and the ureteral wall tone became 3-fold higher as compared to the baseline level. Similar changes were found in the groups of patients that were examined before or after CLT (Fig. 11): the peristalsis amplitude in distal ureter was smaller (0.50 vs 0.81 Ohm), the peristalsis rate was greater (3.3 vs 2.4 min^{-1}), and the tone was higher (6.8 vs 4.7 Ohm^{-1}) after this procedure. In addition, the patients subjected to CLT demonstrated moderately elevated RPP values (18.9±2.6 vs 15.6±1.9 cm H_2O) during the nearest postoperative period (3-7 days). The moderate but persistent RPP increments after endoscopic procedure are supposed to result from malfunction of the distal ureter. In the study using ureteral pressure measurements (Young et al., 2007) it was noted that instrumented human ureter displayed a variable response that appeared to be related to previous physical or pharmacologic effects, and after ureteroscopy peristaltic recovery was variable.

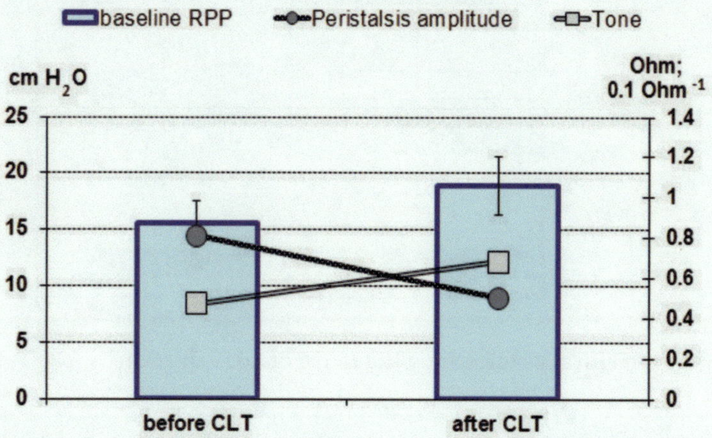

Fig. 11. Functional parameters of UUT urodynamics in patients underwent ureteroscopy (URS) and retrograde contact lithotripsy (CLT)

Thus, the reason of moderately elevated RPP in patients with history of stones for several months as regard to the ureteral function is supposed to concern in strong retrograde contractions, as well as weak contractile activity accompanied by high tone of ureter wall. Lithotripsy procedures are the factors aggravating the changes in RPP and function of ureter in the course of stone disease treatment.

Possible factor responsible for the results of stone elimination during ESWL session can be UUT dilation. The patients that have been subjected to ESWL followed by assessment of its efficacy were divided into three groups according to the range of UUT dilation that preceded this operative procedure (Fig. 12). Then, after lithotripsy session (7-10 day-period), the persistence or restriction of UUT dilation was analysed with respect to ureter functional parameters such as peristalsis amplitude and ureteral wall tone (Fig. 13) evaluated prior to this session.

Successful stone fragmentation and stone-free rate was achieved in 33% patients having no or moderate (<2 cm) UUT dilation, and only in 12% patients with >2 cm UUT dilation. In these patients, the ureteric function was characterized by pronounced retrograde and cystoid contractions (amplitude 1.09±0.14, and 1.11±0.16 Ohm) and moderate or low ureteral wall tone (3.7±0.52, and 0.21±0.01 Ohm^{-1}).

The residual stones after ESWL session were observed in 33% and 70% patients, respectively without UUT dilation, and with >2 cm UUT dilation. These patients' ureteral function was characterized by enhanced ureteral wall tone (9.61±2.52, and 3.10±0.31 Ohm^{-1}) together with pronounced peristalsis amplitude (1.09±0.19, and 1.17±0.09 Ohm). The steinstrasse was observed after ESWL session in 33% patients with no evident UUT dilation whose ureters demonstrated weak peristalsis activity (0.32±0.12 Ohm) and high ureteral wall tone (5.18±2.01 Ohm^{-1}), while the steinstrasse after ESWL session in the cases of dilated UUT, was formed in the patients (20%) whose ureters were characterized by strong ureteral contractions (1.97±0.58 Ohm) and moderate ureteral wall tone (2.08±0.51 Ohm^{-1}).

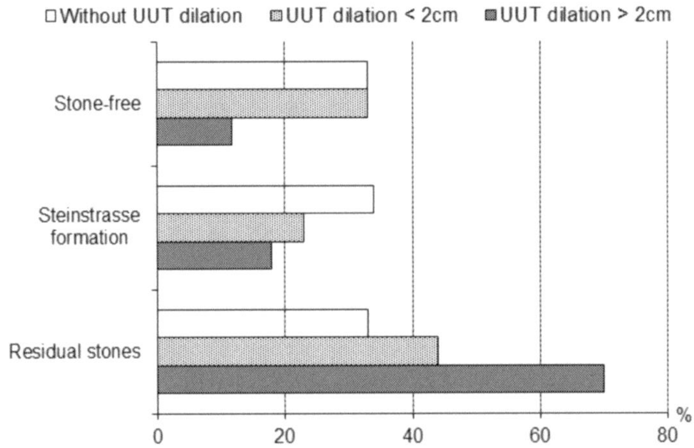

Fig. 12. ESWL session efficacy concerning the range of UUT dilation

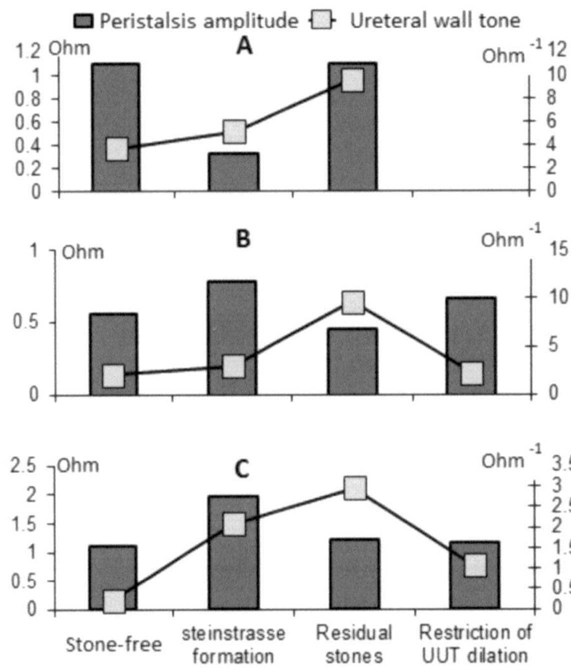

Fig. 13. Interrelation between the efficacy of a single ESWL session and UUT urodynamic status manifested by UUT dilation, and the ureteral functional characteristics. A- without UUT dilation; B- UUT dilation <2 cm; C- UUT dilation >2 cm

Thus, the ureteral function as well as UUT dilation are the important factors influencing stone elimination. In the patients with dilated UUT, the high amplitude of contractions can favor preservation of residual stones or contribute to steinstrasse formation promoting retrograde overshoot of the stone fragments into ureter and renal pelvis after lithotripsy (Fig. 13, C). Less efficacy of ESWL session in these patients with pronounced UUT dilation, and steinstrasse formation despite strong contractile function of their ureter can be explained by possibility of hydrodynamic transmission of ureteral contractions in both upstream and downstream directions along the dilated and opened UUT. These results are well explained on the basis of peristaltic and diuretic mode of urine transport. It is known that during basal hydration, the process of renal pelvic filling and emptying is active, being characterised with the rhythmic pelvic contractions while stimulated diuresis triggers transition from an active to passive peristalsis mode accompanied by transmission of voiding pressures and spontaneous bladder pressures to the kidney.

So, the strong ureteral contractile activity contributed to successful stone elimination in the patients with no (33%) or moderate (33%) UUT dilation, but it accompanied the residual stone formation in the most of patients with dilated (>2 cm) UUT (70%), and in 33% patients with non-dilated UUT.

In the patients with no evident UUT dilation, the strong ureteral contractile activity promoted successful elimination of the stone fragments in the cases of low ureteral wall tone, but also accompanied the residual stone formation in the cases of elevated ureteral wall tone (Fig. 13, A). In both urodynamic conditions relating to UUT dilation, the disorders in vigorous contractile activity manifested by retrograde peristalsis clearly indicated inefficacy of stone fragments elimination treatment.

So, UUT dilation and ureteral mode of peristalsis can influence the stone free-rate after lithotripsy treatment. UUT dilation moderated pronouncedly after successful stone destruction in a 10-day period in the patients characterized with prevalence of strong antegrade contractions (1.68±1.17 Ohm), while US and X-ray picture was worse in those patients who demonstrated depressed contractile activity (0.47±1.14 Ohm), and dilation did not change after stone removal in the patient with aberrant (amplitude 0.08 Ohm) peristalsis evidencing functionally decompensated ureter. We can speculate that ureteric activity is essential for restoring UUT size after treatment while the normal contractile function of ureter can compensate the urodynamic disorders provoked by the stone.

7. Effect of stents on ureteral performance

Our observations of the effects of ureteral stent on the course of stone disease are based on evaluation the parameters of ureteral peristalsis in ureters immediately after being stented. Quantitative and qualitative parameters were measured in 10 patients (16 ureters) examined in dynamics, i.e. before stent indwelling and after its removing. These patients had stone disease complicated by hydronephrosis. In addition, ureters of 10 patients were examined by MIUG during ureteroscopic stent removal after clinically defined period of stent indwelling. On the whole, the effects of ureteral stenting on the ureteral peristalsis were greatly individual.

The individual mode of ureteric peristalsis depended on foregoing pathologic conditions. Analysis of the dynamic changes of ureteral peristalsis in the patients examined before stent insertion and after it withdrawn yielded some important inferences. On the whole, positive effects of ureteral stenting on urodynamic appearance were manifested with UUT dilation restriction. This effect was achieved because the procedure of stent indwelling normalized the peristalsis order and decreased the amplitude of ureteral peristalsis and the ureteral wall tone (Fig. 14). The contractile waves with pronounced slow tonic component (A) became smaller than those before stenting and free from tonic component (As). In one month after stent indwelling, the retrograde and frequent contractile waves (B) lessened (Bs). In patients with local peristaltic abnormalities manifested by irregular contractile activity in various ureteral segments, the stent indwelling corrected the direction of ureteral peristalsis, harmonized ureteral contractions, and moderated the local peristaltic disorders.

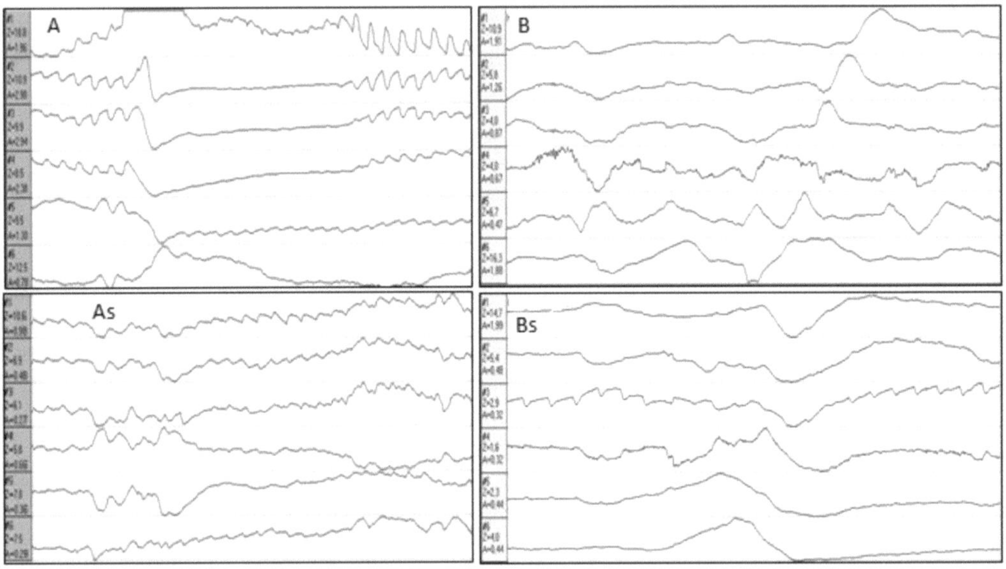

Fig. 14. Examples of ureteral peristalsis demonstrating dynamic changes after internal stenting in two patients (A, and B). A, B- records before stent indwelling; As, Bs- records immediately after stent removing; each record time is 20 sec

In the group of patients examined dynamically, the intrinsic individual mode of ureteral peristalsis preserved its original appearance, and the characteristics of ureteric function did not change significantly during the observed 1-1.5-month period of stenting. At the same time, the peristalsis amplitude and ureteral wall tone decreased in the most of patients (80%). In a small group of patients (20%), the stent indwelling augmented the ureteral peristaltsis.

In the group of patients examined only once immediately after 1-1.5-months stent indwelling by MIUG, the strong peristalsis amplitude (1.24±0.16 Ohm) and low ureteral wall tone (2.22±0.63 Ohm^{-1}) was recorded in 5 of 10 patients observed. The rest 5 patients demonstrated weak aberrant peristalsis (0.20±0.04 Ohm) and high ureteral wall tone (6.34±1.08 Ohm^{-1}). The observed peristalsis characteristics may reflect different individual ureteral conditions, and different reactions to stenting.

MIUG recordings illustrate the irritation of ureteral wall after stent indwelling manifested by frequent arrhythmic bursts of bioelectrical activity that appeared periodically in various parts of the ureter. We can suppose that the stent itself acts like a stone and irritates the ureter wall stimulating the contractile activity of smooth muscles. Some ureters can react to stent indwelling by increased ureteral contractions and demonstrate hyperfunction (fig.15, A). However, some ureters are unable to respond to foreign body insertion with increased peristalsis amplitude and remained decompensated (B).

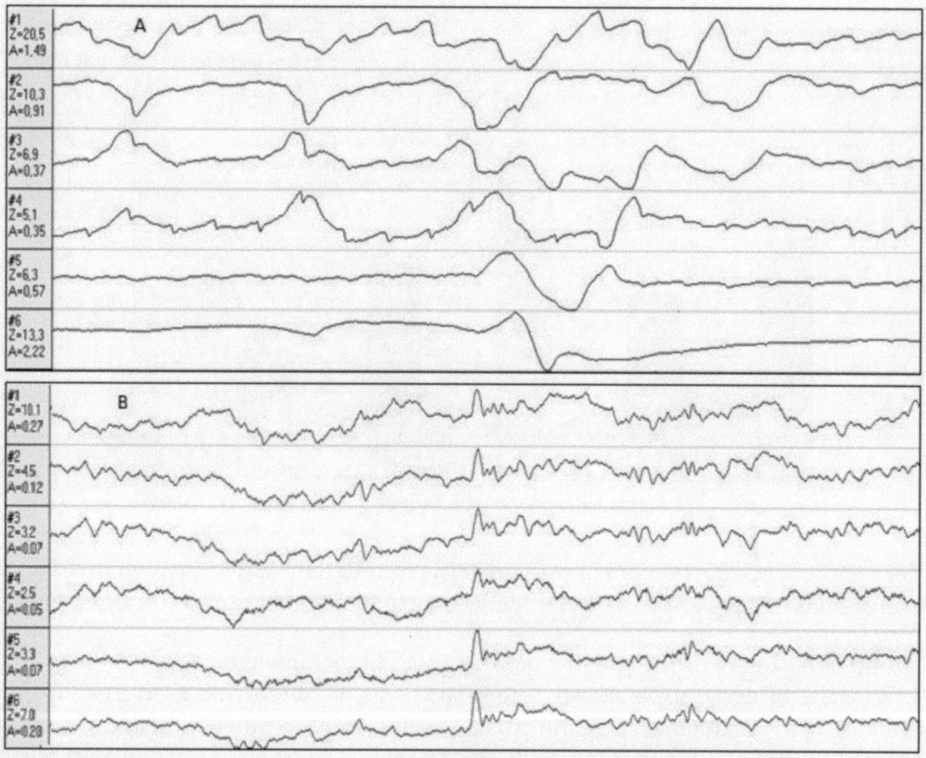

Fig. 15. Examples of ureteral peristalsis after internal stenting obtained by MIUG in two patients: A- with strong contractile activity in the ureter, and B- with weak peristalsis; each record time is 20 sec

There are still controversial opinions on the necessity of stent indwelling and corresponding indications for ureteral stenting for the patients subjected to ureteroscopy and lithotripsy (Venkatesh et al., 2005; Haleblian et al., 2008). Clinical examinations of the patients did not reveal any difference in the results of stent indwelling despite the differences in the character of the contractile function manifested by pronounced or aberrant peristalsis. In our opinion, the relief of UUT obstructive symptoms, and stabilization or improvement of renal function after stent indwelling is a likely outcome of stenting. These results were frequently observed in patients demonstrating elimination or moderation of local peristaltic disorders, the uniform peristaltic activity of ureteric regions.

The peristalsis of all ureter regions in patient with ureteropelvic junction obstruction and concomitant caluli (Fig. 16) was monitored in the 1-st City Hospital before simultaneous stone and stricture removal following by stent insertion. The pronounced peristalsis was recorded in renal pelvis above stricture region, and in middle ureter (0.88-1.15 Ohm). However, the peristaltic waves spread in opposite directions: they were constantly retrograde above the stricture region and obtained antegrade and cystoid character in the lower ureter regions. In this patient, functional peristaltic disorders were reversible, and positive results of treatment were achieved according HUN resolution and renal function restoration.

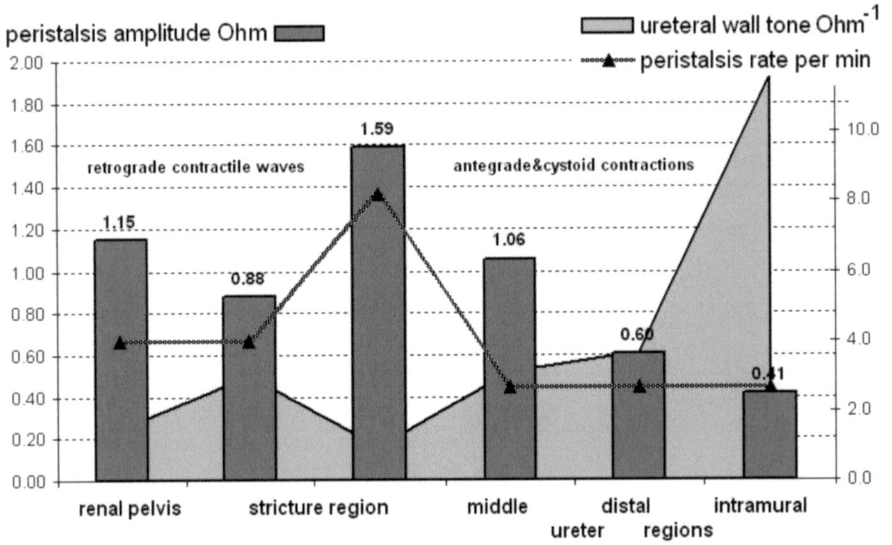

Fig. 16. Functional characteristics of the peristalsis recorded by MIUG method in different ureteral regions of a patient with ureteropelvic junction obstruction and concomitant caluli

The group of hydronephrotic patients (n=5) with UPJ strictures were analysed according to the parameters of ureteral peristalsis before stricture correction, and then in a 10-14 days after endoscopic treatment and immediately after stent removal (Fig. 17). Successful endoscopic treatment was marked with the following positive urodynamic changes: 1) previously reduced mean peristalsis amplitude of dilated renal pelvis and ureter increased, 2) initially high peristaltic frequency above stricture region decreased, and 3) pronounced ureteral wall tone dropped.

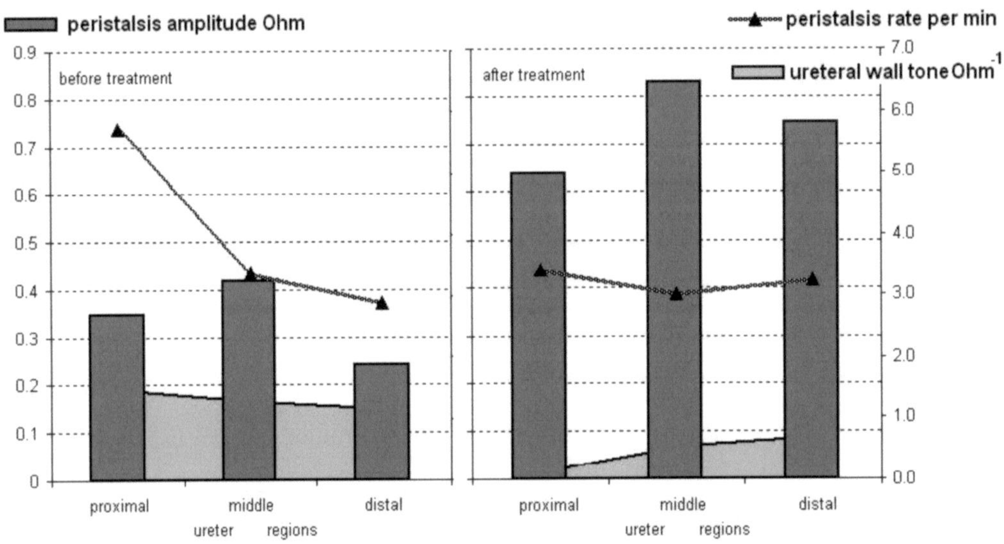

Fig. 17. Changes in ureteral function obtained with MIUG after endoscopic UPJ stricture correction and stenting in patients with hydronephrosis

When the urodynamic data obtained during the course of treatment corroborated such tendency and if the quantitative characteristics of ureteric contractile function became more uniform in different ureteral parts after the treatment, the correction was considered as successful. It was clinically approved. Moreover, qualitative features of ureteral peristalsis tended to be in order (Fig. 18): the amount of retrograde, cystoid, and aberrant arrhythmic contractile waves diminished, while normal antegrade contractions were more often observed along the ureter than before endoscopic stricture correction and stent indwelling.

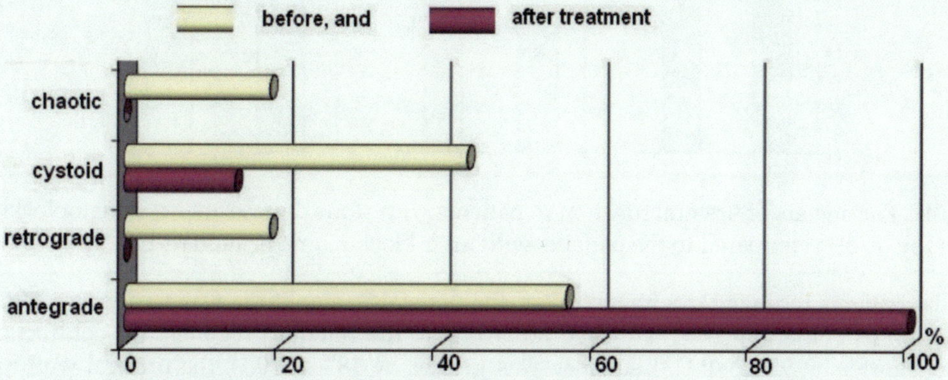

Fig. 18. Character of ureteral peristaltic waves obtained with MIUG after endoscopic UPJ stricture correction and stenting in patients with hydronephrosis

So, in hydronephrosis, the positive urodynamic changes resulted from successful treatment are the concordant uniform peristaltic activity in all ureteric regions, an increment of the amplitude of ureter contractions, a decrease in the ureteral wall tone, and a drop in the peristaltic rate, especially in the upper region of the ureter. In these cases, the signs of peristaltic orientation disorders and arrhythmia diminished.

Thus, stenting per se can be helpful to harmonization of peristaltic process in dilated ureter and reversion of the abnormal hydronephrotic changes if the intrinsic contractile compensatory reserves are safe. In so going, the normalization process might be indicative on the functional changes in the examined UUT not accompanied by severe structural lesions.

8. Peculiarities of ureteral function in patients with stones in the upper urinary tract after alpha-blocking medication

In this study, the parameters of the ureteral peristalsis and RPP values were compared in two groups of patients, respectively, who were treated with α-adrenoblocker tamsulosin (0.4 mg daily) in addition to the standard regimen, and patients without α-blocking medication. Patients in both groups (15 and 25 persons, consequently) were matched according to the size and location of the stones in UUT.

The positive effects of α-blocking were demonstrated in clinical settings with varying rate of success and the mechanism of this therapy was analyzed. In ureteral pressure measurements, a hypothesis has been advanced that reduction in pressure generation may be an essential factor promoting stone passage during α-adrenoblocking therapy

(Davenport et al., 2007). Moreover, it was suggested that these drugs work by preventing an augmented uncoordinated muscular activity whilst maintaining peristalsis, thereby promoting stone passage. Our data corroborate this hypothesis (Fig. 19).

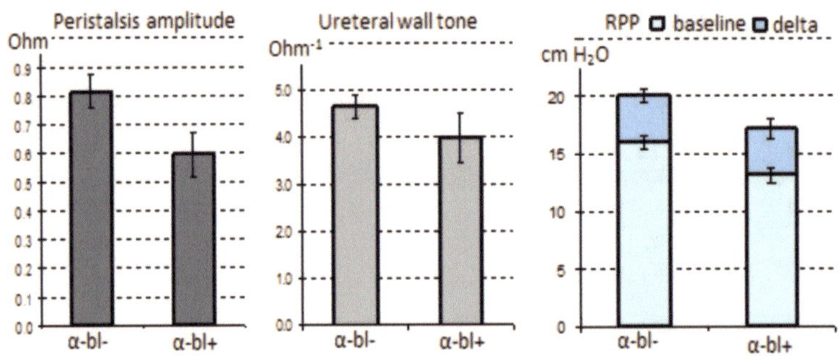

Fig. 19. Parameters of ureteral function in patients with stone disease after α-adrenoblocking therapy (α-bl+) compared to the patients without α-blocking medication (α-bl-)

In the patients receiving α-adrenoblocker, the peristalsis amplitude was weaker by 2.9±3.5 Ohm ($p<0.02$) than in patients treated according to the standard regimen, the contractions were shorter by 9% ($p<0.1$), frequency was greater by 18% ($p<0.1$), the ureteral wall tone was smaller by 14% ($p<0.5$), and the normal antegrade regular contractions were more frequently (by 30%) observed. The average RPP values were smaller by 15-28% after α-adrenoblocking therapy, although diuresis via nephrostomy tubes was similar in both groups (1.1±0.1 and 0.9±0.1 ml/min).

Moreover, different urodynamic changes were found after α-adrenoblocking therapy in patients with proximal and distal stones in UUT (Fig. 20). In the patients with stones located in the kidney and proximal ureter, there were no significant differences in the parameters of ureteral peristalsis between the examined groups except for the lower peristalsis amplitude by 38% ($p<0.02$) in the patients receiving α-adrenoblocker medication, and there was no intergroup difference in RPP. While in the patients with distal ureteral stones, no differences were found between the parameters of peristalsis in both groups, but RPP value was significantly smaller in the patients receiving α-adrenoblocking therapy. The baseline and peristaltic pressure was smaller in this group by, respectively, 47% and 39% compared to the patients treated according only to the standard regimen.

As discussed in the above, differently located stones in UUT could evoke different reflexes, and, therefore, different functional urodynamic changes. In view of the dominant role of adrenoreceptors in ureteral function modulation, α-adrenoblocking therapy can induce urodynamic changes by this pathway. Thus, we can suppose that the renal and proximal ureteral stones can evoke reflex irritation of the excitatory adrenergic fibers in distal ureter that stimulate its contractions; therefore, α-adrenoblocker can moderate the ureteral contractions by blocking adrenergic receptors. Elevated RPP in patients with proximal stones in UUT is urodynamic in nature, i.e., it predominantly results from obstruction with a stone hindering urine outflow from the kidney. Therefore, α-adrenoblocker could not affect this parameter. In the case of distal stones, irritation of distal ureter via adrenergic excitatory mechanism can induce reflex elevation of pressure in kidney; therefore, α-adrenoblocker can induce reduction in RPP by blocking corresponding receptors.

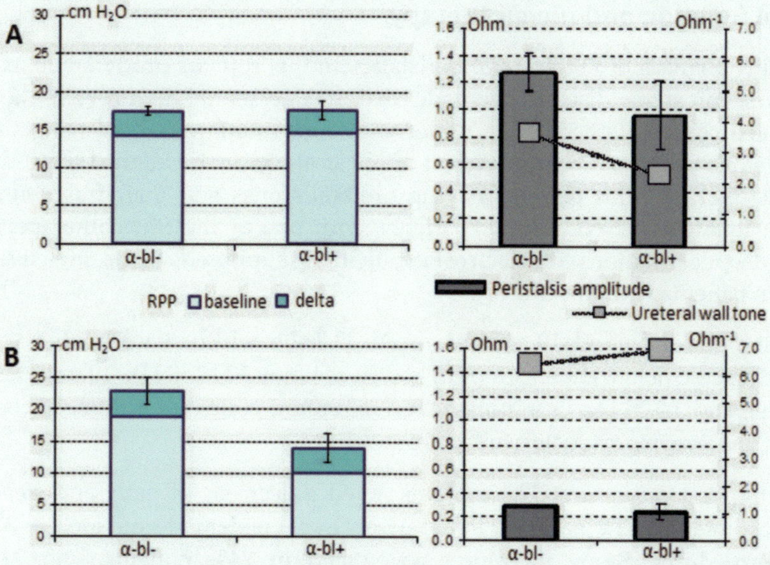

Fig. 20. Different effects of α-adrenoblocking therapy in patients with stones in kidney and proximal ureter (A), and with distal ureteral stones (B)

Individual ureteral peristalsis peculiarities mentioned above, such as pronounced contractile activity, or aberrant peristalsis, also can impress α-adrenoblocking effects on ureteric function. The patients whose ureters demonstrate aberrant peristalsis, i.e. very weak chaotic waves and high ureteral wall tone cannot response well to α-adrenoblocking therapy. We suppose that such aberrant peristalsis can result from previous general inflammatory and fibrotic changes in ureteral wall that cannot be modulated by autonomic neural influences. There were no differences between the parameters of ureteral peristalsis in such patients with or without α-adrenoblocking therapy. Their ureters do not actively participate in urine transport by peristaltic activity, urine transport in these patients is fulfilled under pressure gradient like as during diuretic flow, and therefore such ureters need to be treated by creating unobstructed low-pressure urine passage.

When patients with adequate peristaltic function were compared, the peristalsis amplitude was smaller in the patients receiving α-adrenoblocker compared to that without this medication (0.97±0.25 vs 1.30±0.14 Ohm), the ureteral wall tone was lower (2.30±0.55 vs 3.60±0.56 Ohm^{-1}), the contractions were shorter by 17% and faster by 52%, and RPP was smaller (13.50±0.69 vs 22.90±5.40 cm H_2O) indicating the better urine drainage from the kidney.

Thus, efficacy of α-adrenoblocker treatment can be achieved for different stone location in the upper urinary tract, but it largely depends on the individual ureter status. In patients with functional peristaltic disorders, especially with those provoked by increased adrenergic stimulation, treatment with α-adrenoblockers would be helpful in the terms of contractility normalization and ureteral wall relaxation. However, pronounced organic changes in ureteral wall caused by previous inflammatory or fibrotic processes characterized by aberrant peristalsis can be responsible for medication inefficacy.

9. Ureteral function and physiotherapy

The foregoing analysis of the ureteral peristalsis and its role for urodynamic manifestation in the course of stone disease persuade that it is essential to prevent the increased, uncoordinated contractile activity in ureter whilst maintaining normal peristalsis, thereby promoting stone passage. The application of physical factors broadened the indications for conservative therapy with patients having ureteral stones and their fragments including stainstrasse following ESWL. Our experience with one of the physiotherapeutic method based on deep oscillations of electrostatic field is supposed to be effective for stone expulsion in patients with urolithiasis.

The clinical study included 19 patients aged 39.7±4.6 which were treated with various pulsed electrostatic field frequencies (I, II, and III regime): 120-180 Hz (10 minutes), 65-85 Hz (10 minutes), and 14-25 Hz (5 minutes). The minimum course of treatment consisted of 2 procedures, the maximum - consisted of 7 procedures.

Following the first procedure, 32% patients noted a decrease of pain, and steady diuresis increase was noted in 42% patients. Renal parenchyma oedema terminated in 37% patients after 3-5 procedures. Stone migration was noted in 74% patients, and 21% patients experienced renal colic attacks with the successive spontaneous stone passage (Fig.21). Concrement elimination has made up 86% with stones ≤5 mm; 73% with stones 5-10 mm; and 83% with steinstrasse length up to 10 mm. One patient was excluded from the study because of pyelonephritis attack development following the first procedure. On the whole, the treatment had no effect on the recovery in 21% patients.

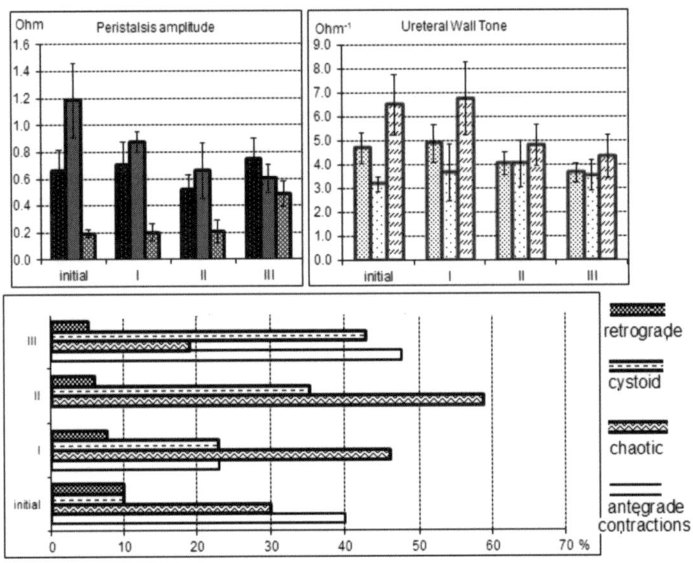

Fig. 21. Distribution of patients with stone disease according to clinical effects of physiotherapy

Concerning these favouring clinical results, acute effects of this physiotherapy on ureteral function were assessed for 8 patients undergoing ureteroscopy by MIUG method. Two external electrodes were applied on the front abdominal wall in projection of ureter, and diagnostic probe was installed into a distal ureter. The ureteral peristalsis has been monitoring during 3-minute period initially, and then within each physiotherapeutic regime.

The overt effects of examined physical factors were documented by immediate changes in peristalsis amplitude, peristalsis rate, ureteral wall tone, and the character and direction of contractile waves travelling along the ureter. These parameters of ureteric contractile function changed individually in patients depending on the frequency of applied electrostatic field and initial ureter status (Fig.22).

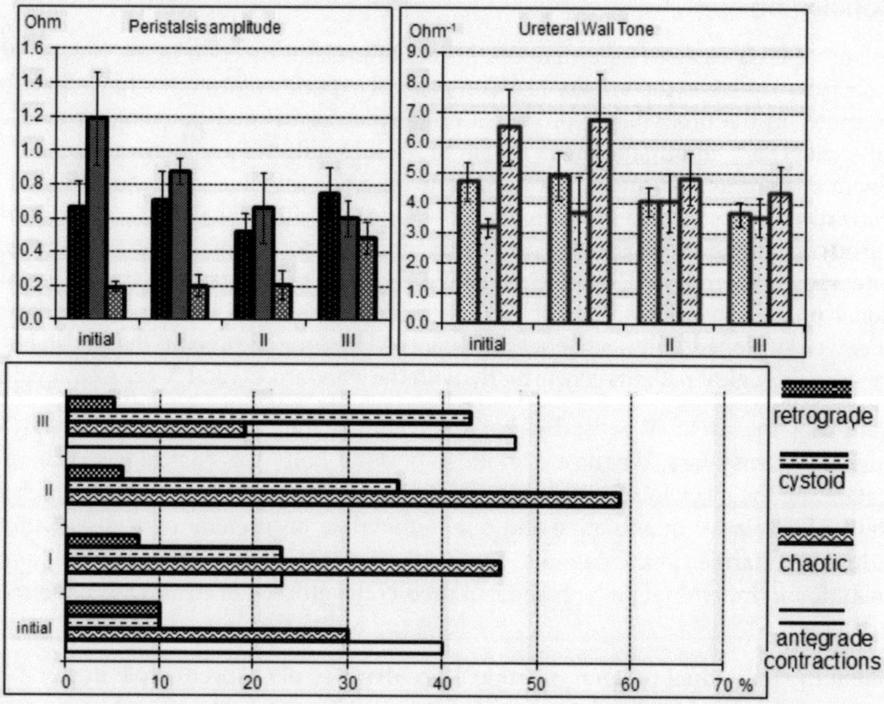

Fig. 22. Dynamic changes in the peristalsis amplitude, ureteral wall tone, and contractile wave characteristics within three (I, II, and III) applied physiotherapeutic regimes. Consecutive columns describe the changes in peristalsis amplitude and ureteral wall tone in different patient groups, respectively, all 8 patients examined, patients with initially strong contractile activity in ureter, and patients with aberrant ureteral peristalsis

On the whole, peristalsis rate increased at all frequencies by 30-50%. The ureteral wall tone decreased by 14% and 22% ($p<0.001$) in response to electrostatic oscillations at frequencies 85 and 180 Hz, respectively. The chaotic contractions frequently (30%) observed prior to physiotherapy were replaced by antegrade (48%) or cystoid (43%) peristalsis accompanied by an inhibition of retrograde contractions. No average significant changes were noted for the peristalsis amplitude, however, it has been changing depending on initial conditions with individual patients. The strong initially contractions used to decrease after physiotherapeutic stimulation, while weak contractile activity used to enhance in patients with aberrant peristalsis.

These findings suggest that physiotherapy is capable to affect the ureteral contractile function by normalizing the character of its peristalsis, decreasing ureteral wall tone, and individually stimulating the weak ureteral contractions or decreasing strong retrograde contractile waves. The energy of deep oscillation with electrostatic field can induce changes evidencing to spasmolitic, and diuretic effects of this procedure. In complex lithokinetic therapy of patients with stone disease, physiotherapy can be helpful in facilitating stone evacuation, and restoration of urine passage due to improved diuresis. It is likely this procedure in some cases can replace medication.

10. Conclusion

Physiology of UUT established an important role of ureteral function in the process of urine transport from kidney to the urinary bladder. A lot of experimental studies have described the role of ureter in the urodynamic processes under the normal and pathologic conditions. In clinical settings, less information is available to reliably reflect the ureter function relating to urodynamic disorders because the technique is still invasive and necessitates ureter catheterization. Despite these instrumental difficulties, the functional urodynamic studies on UUT urodynamics have been carried out in patients with stone disease using the intraluminal pressure measurements and videourodynamic technique. At present vital importance of functional urodynamic diagnostics of UUT is evident. Based on numerous experiments on animals, we developed a multichannel impedance technique to observe the peristalsis along the ureter in urological patients concurrently with the standard US and X-ray examinations.

Evaluation of the ureteral peristalsis by multichannel impedance ureterography (MIUG) provides supplementary diagnostic tools important both for clinical practice and for understanding the mechanisms of urodynamic disorders in patients with stone disease. This method yields relative quantitative and qualitative data on ureteral peristalsis and reveals individual peculiarities in the patients. This method can be useful when choosing a medical treatment for an individual patient, and can predict the efficacy of treatment in the course of stone disease.

Undoubtedly, individual ureteral functional peculiarities play specific role in stone disease course, and they must be taken into consideration in the course of treatment.

The strong contractile activity can play the double role in the process of stone passage after ESWL. It was shown to be a facilitating factor, if contractions spread antegradely towards a bladder through the dilated or undilated UUT. But in the dilated UUT, complications like residual stone fragments and steinstrasse formation are quite possible, especially in case of strong retrograde and uncoordinated contractions.

Strong contractile activity in ureter is often observed in primary patients. This activity even being functionally destroyed can be easily modulated by medication, and can be reversible after emergent stone removal. But strong persistent retrograde contractions may cause urine refluxes and stagnation complicated by inflammation.

Weak contractile activity was a characteristic of ureter inherent for lot of patients with stone disease. Such aberrant peristalsis was frequently seen in patients with long history of stones in UUT. Also, aberrant peristalsis and high ureteral wall tone was observed in place of the stone or stricture location. Patients with such mode of peristalsis usually need long period to rehabilitate the UUT urodynamics after lithotripsy procedures. Stents might be helpful in treatment of the peristalsis disorders in dilated UUT.

The quantitative parameters of UUT peristalsis obtained by MIUG that give worse treatment results in combination with the qualitative features are:

- weak UUT peristaltic activity + high ureteral wall tone,
- strong ureteral contractions + retrograde peristaltic waves.

These ureteral functional characteristics are shown to be the reason of RPP elevation evidencing to inadequate renal drainage.

The renal pelvis pressure is a complex urodynamic parameter. A lot of factors are responsible for RPP elevation that would produce a harmful effect on renal function. There are no doubts that the main players here are obstruction and inflammation. The quicker removal of obstruction and rapid elimination of inflammation mean better restoration of pelvic pressure. Also, elevation in interstitial pressure due to continuing pathologic process in renal parenchyma, and inadequate ureteral function that must provide urine outflow from kidney can be additional factors responsible for moderately increased pressure in renal pelvis after elimination of the main factors.

Thus, ureteral peristalsis and RPP are valuable indicators of functional UUT urodynamic disorders. Assessment of these functional parameters in different patients under various clinical situations persuades us that except the general changes typical of disease and treatment modality, the individual functional features are attended anytime and anywhere. Therefore, the parameters of ureteral function and pressure in renal pelvis are likely to be controlled in the course of disease. Individual evaluation of these UUT urodynamic characteristics might be useful in definition whether patient will respond to medication and conservative treatment, or more invasive management is indicated.

11. Acknowledgment

We are indebted to many people for their help with the complex urodynamic examination of patients with stone disease upon which this article is based. We would like to thank Mr. Martov Aleksey G., Mr. Moskalenko Sergey A., Mr. Fachretdinov Gennadiy. of the Moscow Urological City Hospital N. 47, and Mr. Dzeranov Nikolay K. & Mr. Beshliev Djamal A. of the Moscow Research Institute of Urology in whose departments the major part of this work was carried out. On the technical side I am grateful to Mr. Revenko Sergey V. who has given me encouragement, advice, and invaluable assistance.

12. References

Airik, R., Trowe, M.-O., Foik, A., Farin, H.F., Petry, M., Schuster-Gossler, K., Schweizer, M., Scherer, G., Kist, R. & Kispert, A. (2010). Hydroureternephrosis due to loss of Sox9-regulated smooth muscle cell differentiation of the ureteric mesenchyme. *Human Molecular Genetics*, Vol. 19, N. 24, pp. 4918–4929

Constantinou, C.E. & Yamaguchi, O. (1981). Multiple-coupled pacemaker system in renal pelvis of the unicalyceal kidney. *American Journal of Physiology*, Vol. 241, pp. R412–R418

Constantinou, C.E. (1974). Renal pelvic pacemaker control of ureteral peristaltic rate. *American Journal of Physiology*, Vol. 226, pp. 1413–1419

Davenport, K., Timoney, A.G. & Keeley, F.X. (2006). A comparative in vitro study to determine the beneficial effect of calcium-channel and alpha (1)-adrenoceptor antagonism on human ureteric activity. *British Journal of Urology International*, Vol. 98, pp. 651-655

Davenport, K., Timoney, A.G. & Keeley, F.X. (2007). The Role of Ureteral Relaxation in the Promotion of Stone Passage. *CP900, Renal Stone Disease, 1" Annual International Urolithiasis Research Symposium*, edited by A. P. Evan, J. E. Lingeman, and J. C. Williams, Jr. 2007 American Institute of Physics 978-0-7354-0406-9/07, pp. 243-252

Davenport, K. & Keeley, F.X. (2011). Medical Expulsive Therapy. *Urinary Tract Stone Disease*, Part 10, pp. 651-658

Davis, D.M. (1954). The Hydrodynamics of the Upper Urinary Tract. *Annals of Surgery*, Vol. 140, N. 6, pp. 839-849

Dwyer, T.M. & Schmidt-Nielsen, B. (2003). The renal pelvis: machinery that concentrates urine in the papilla. *News in Physiological Sciences*, Vol.18, pp.1-6

Grampsas, S.A., Chandhoke, P.S., Fan, J., Glass, M.A., Townsend, R., Johnson, A.M. & Gabow, P. (2000). Anatomic and metabolic risk factors for nephrolithiasis in patients with autosomal dominant polycystic kidney disease. *American Journal of Kidney Diseases*, Vol. 36, pp. 53-57

Grisk, O., Packebusch, M., Antje, C., Steinbach, T.S., Kopp, U.C. & Rettig, R. (2010). Endothelin-1-induced activation of rat renal pelvic contractions depends on cyclooxygenase-1 and Rho kinase. *AJP - ReguPhysiol*, Vol. 299, N. 6, pp. R1602-R1609

Haleblian, G., Kijvikai, K., de la Rosette, J. & Preminger, G. (2008). Ureteral Stenting and Urinary Stone Management: A Systematic Review. *Journal of Urology*, Vol.179, pp. 424-430

Hannappel, J. & Golenhofen, K. (1974). The effect of catecholamines on ureteral peristalsis in different species (dog, guinea-pig and rat). Pflügers Archiv European Journal of Physiology, Vol. 350, N. 1, pp.55-68

Harada, T., Miyagata, S., Etori, K., Kumasaki, T. & Noto, H. (1984). [Evaluation of the pelvioureteral function through an impedance urine bolus-metry][Article in Japanese]. *Nippon Heikatsukin Gakkai Zasshi*, Vol. 20, N.6, pp. 445-453

Hashitani, H., Lang, R.J., Retsu Mitsui, R., Yoshio Mabuchi, Y. & Suzuki, H. (2009). Distinct effects of CGRP on typical and atypical smooth muscle cells involved in generating spontaneous contractions in the mouse renal pelvis. *British Journal of Pharmacology*, Vol. 158, N. 8, pp. 2030–2045

Husmann, D.A., Milliner, D.S. & Segura, J.V. (1995). Ureteropelvic junction obstruction with a simultaneous renal calculus: long-term followup. *Journal of Urology*, Vol. 153, pp. 1399-1403

Hurtado, R., Bub G. & Herzlinger, D. (2010). The pelvis–kidney junction contains HCN3, a hyperpolarization-activated cation channel that triggers ureter peristalsis. *Kidney International*, Vol. 77, pp. 500-508

Page, J.B., Humphreys, S., Davenport, D., Crispen, P. & Venkatesh, R. (2011). Second prize: In-vivo physiological impact of alpha blockade on the porcine ureter with distal ureteral obstruction. *Journal of Endourology*, Vol. 25, N. 3, pp. 391-396

Jung, H., Frimodt-Møller, P.C., Osther P.J.S. & Mortensen J. (2006). Pharmacological effect on pyeloureteric dynamics with a clinical perspective: a review of the literature. *Urological Research,* Vol. 34, N 6, pp. 341-350

Jung H. & Osther P.J.S. (2011). How high is the intraluminal pelvic pressure during flexible ureterorenoscopy. *European Urology Supplements,* Vol. 10, N 7, pp. 484

Kim, S., Jacob, J.S., Kim, D.C., Rivera, R., Lim, R.P. & Lee, V.S. (2008). Time-resolved dynamic contrast-enhanced MR urography for the evaluation of ureteral peristalsis: initial experience. *Journal of Magnetic Resonance Imaging,* Vol.28, pp. 1293–1298

Kinn, A.C. (1996). Progress in urodynamic research on the upper urinary tract: implications for practical urology. *Urological Research,* Vol.24, N.1, pp.1-7

Kinn, A.C. & Lykkeskov-Andersen, H. (2002). Impact on ureteral peristalsis in a stented ureter. An experimental study in the pig. *Urological Research,* Vol. 30, N. 4, pp. 213-218

Kobayashi M. (1965). Effects of Na and Ca on the generation and conduction of excitation in the ureter, *American Journal of Physiology,* Vol.208, pp. 715-719

Lang, R.J. & Klemm, M.F. (2005). Interstitial cell of Cajal-like cells in the upper urinary tract. *Journal of Cellular and Molecular Meicine,* Vol. 9, pp. 543–556

Lee, H.W., Baak, C.H., Lee, M.Y. & Kim, Y.C. (2011). Spontaneous Contractions Augmented by Cholinergic and Adrenergic Systems in the Human Ureter. *Korean J PhysiolPharmacol,* Vol. 15, N 1, pp. 37–41

Levent, A. & Buyukafsar, K. (2004). Expression of Rho-kinase (ROCK-1 and ROCK-2) and its substantial role in the contractile activity of the sheep ureter. *British Journal of Pharmacology,* Vol.143, pp.431–437

Matin, S.F., & Streem, S.B. (2000). Metabolic risk factors in patients with ureteropelvic junction obstruction and renal calculi. *Journal of Urology,* Vol. 163, pp. 1676-1681

McHale, N.G., Hollywood, M.A., Sergeant, G.P., Shafei1, M., Thornbury, K.T. & Ward S.M. (2006). Organization and function of ICC in the urinary tract. *Journal of Physiology,* Vol. 576, N. 3, pp. 689–694

Mudraya, I.S., Kirpatovsky, V.I., Martov, A.G. & Obuchova T.V. (2001). Contractile Function of Upper Urinary Tract after Indwelling Ureteral Prosthesis: Experimental Investigation . Journal of Endourology, June Vol.15, N.5, pp. 533-539

Mudraya, I.S., Kirpatovsky, V.I. & Martov, A.G. (2007). Bioimpedance Methods in Urology Functional Diagnostics. *IFMBE Proceedings 13th International Conference on Electrical Bioimpedance and the 8th Conference on Electrical Impedance Tomography ICEBI,* August 29th - September 2nd 2007, Graz, Austria 10.1007/978-3-540-73841-1_182

Mudraya, I.S. & Khodyreva, L.A. (2011). The role of functional urodynamic disorders in the pathogenesis of urolithiasis". *Archivio Italiano di Urologia e Andrologia,* Vol. 83, N 1, pp. 31-36

Notley (1971). The innervation and musculature of the human ureter. *Annals of the Royal College of Surgeons of England,* Vol. 49, pp. 250-267

Pezzone, M.A., Watkins, S.C., Alber, S.M., King, W.E., de Groat, W.C., Chancellor, M.B. & Fraser, M.O. (2003). Identification of c-kit-positive cells in the mouse ureter: the interstitial cells of Cajal of the urinary tract. *American Journal of Physiology Renal Physiology,* Vol. 284, pp. 925–929

Pick, D.L., Shelkovnikov, S., Kaplan A.G., Louie, M.K., Purdy, R., McDougall, E.M. & Clayman, R.V. (2011). A Novel Ex-Vivo Ureteral Apparatus for Assessing the

Impact of Intraluminal Pharmaceutical Agents on Ureteral Physiology. *Journal of Endourology*, Vol, 25, N 4, pp. 681-685

Rasidovic D., Kearney, D., Boyle, K.-M. & Bund, S.J. (2010). The assessment of rat ureteral pressure generation in vitro: regional heterogeneity and influence of distending pressure. *Acta Physiologica Hungarica*, Vol. 97, N. 3, pp. 307-315

Rose, J. G. & Gillenwater, J.Y. (1973). Pathophysiology of ureteral obstruction. American Journal of Physiology, Vol. 225, pp. 830-837

Roshani, H., Dabhoiwala, N.F., Tee, S., Dijkhuis, T., Kurth, K.H., Ongerboer de Visser, B.W., de Jong, J.M. & Lamers, W.H. (1999). A study of ureteric peristalsis using a single catheter to record EMG, impedance, and pressure changes. *Techniques in Urology*, Vol.5, N.1, pp. 61-66

Roshani, H., Dabhoiwala, N.F., Dijkhuis, T., Ongerboer de Visser, B.W., Kurth, K.H. & Lamers, W.H. (2000). An electro-myographic study of the distal porcine ureter. *The Journal of Urology*, Vol. 163, N.5, pp. 1570-1576

Roshani, H., Dabhoiwala, N.F., Dijkhuis, T. & Lamers, W.H. (2002). Intraluminal pressure changes in vivo in the middle and distal pig ureter during propagation of a peristaltic wave. *Urology*, Vol.59, N2, pp. 298-302

Roshani, H., Dabhoiwala, N.F., Dijkhuis, T., Pfaffendorf, M., Boon, T. & Lamers, W.H. (2003). Pharmacological Modulation of Ureteral Peristalsis in a Chronically Instrumented Conscious Pig Model. I: Effect of Cholinergic Stimulation and Inhibition. *The Journal of Urology*, Vol. 170, N. 1, pp. 264-267

Santicioli, P. & Maggi, C.A. (1998). Myogenic and neurogenic factors in the control of pyeloureteral motility and ureteral peristalsis. *Pharmacological Reviews*, Vol. 50, N 4, pp. 683–721

Shafik, A. (1996). Electroureterogram: human study of the electromechanical activity of the ureter. *Urology*, Vol. 48, pp. 696–699

Shafik, A. (1998). Ureteric profilometry. A study of the ureteric pressure profile in the normal and pathologic ureter. *Scandinavian Journal of Urology and Nephrology*, Vol. 32, N.1, pp. 14-19

Sorensen, C.M. & Chandhoke, P.S. (2002). Is lower pole caliceal anatomy predictive of extracorporeal shock wave lithotripsy success for primary lower pole kidney stones? *Journal of Urology*. Vol.168. N6, pp. 2377-2382

Tindall, A. R. (1972) . Preliminary Observations on the Mechanical and electrical activity of the Rat Ureter. *Journal of Physiology*, Vol. 223, pp. 633-647

Venkatesh, R., Landman, J., Minor, S.D., Lee, D.I., Rehman, J., Vanlangendonck, R., Ragab, M., Morrissey, K., Sundaram, C. P. & Clayman R.V. (2005). Impact of a Double-Pigtail Stent on Ureteral Peristalsis in the Porcine Model: Initial Studies Using a Novel Implantable Magnetic Sensor. *Journal of Endourology*, March 1, Vol. 19, N. 2, pp. 170-176

Weiss, R.M., Tamarkin, F.J. & Wheeler, M.A. (2006). Pacemaker activity in the upper urinary tract. *Journal of Smooth Muscle Research*, Vol. 42, N. 4, pp. 103–115

Young, A.J., Acher, P.L., Lynn, B., McCahy, P.J. & Miller, R.A. (2007). Evaluation of novel technique for studying ureteral function in vivo. *Journal of Endourology*, Vol. 21, N. 1, pp. 94-99

6

Prevention of Bladder Tumor Recurrence

Shapiro Amos and Ofer N. Gofrit
The Department of Urology, Hadassah University Hospital, Jerusalem, Israel

The Way to Prevent Tumor Impantation is by Washing out the Cancer Cells and Prevent Its Addherence Prevention of Tumor Recurrence After Transurethral Resection by Means of Bladder Irrigation with Distilled Water - A Prospective Randomized Study with a Long-Term Follow-up.

1. Introduction

Superficial papillary tumors of the bladder recur in about 70% of patients in the first 2 years following treatment by transe urethral resection (TUR). Since there is no other evidence of mucosal changes in random biopsies it seems that the high recurrence rate is due to tumor implantation. We tried to find out whether irrigation with distilled water of the bladder following TUR will reduce tumor recurrence.

2. Material and methods

Sixty nine patients were enlisted for a prospective randomized controlled study in order to investigate the efficacy of bladder irrigation with distilled water for 24 hours following a transurethral resection of first time papillary transitional cell tumors of the urinary bladder. These patients were compared to a group of patients that were not irrigated at all. There were 31 patients in the first group and 38 in the control. All patients had grade 2 transitional cell tumors (average 1.2 tumors per patient). Random biopsies that were taken at the time of operation showed no additional pathology.

3. Results

In the irrigated group there were 8 (25%) recurrences in the first 24 months of follow-up while at the same period of time there were 22 (58%) recurrences in the control group, $p=0.007$ (using a chi square analysis). On longer follow-up of between 2 to 10 years (mean 6 years) there was no difference in tumor appearance between the two groups 8 out of 23 (37%) in the irrigated group and 5 out of 16 (31%) in the remaining patients in the control group, $p=0.6119$ using the same statistical tool. The recurrence rate of low-grade superficial papillary tumor of the bladder is about 70% (1). Most of the recurrences occur in the first year after the tran-urethral tumor resection (TUR) and 95% of the recurrence occur within two years after the resection (2). Although this is a low grade malignant tumor and biopsies that are taken randomly at the time of the resection are normal, the tumor shows a high tendency to recur, and this observation needs some sort of biological explanation. The tumors tend to occur at the bladder neck where the resectoscope most frequently injures the normal mucosa and at the dome of the bladder where distention of the bladder while inflating it during the operation tends to crack the epithelial lining. During transurethral-resection of a bladder tumor many viable malignant cells are floating free in the bladder and have the capability of adhering to a raw surface in the bladder (3). These two facts lead to the idea that the recurrence is iatrogenic: meaning that cells that were floating in the bladder during the TUR are implanted into the injured bladder mucosa. If this hypothesis is correct then elimination of the viable cells and disabling of the adhesive properties of the cells should significantly lower the recurrence rate of this tumor. Distilled water irrigation of the bladder should reach these goals. In order to prove this hypothesis a controlled randomized study was conducted from 1983 until 1990 in which the efficacy of washing the bladder with 12 liters of water in 24h was compared to no irrigation during the post operative period. Tumor occurrences were compared in these two groups at the end of the first two years and from then on.

4. Patients selection

Eighty four patients entered the study, 15 had high grade tumors or carcinoma in situ and the were treated right away with Bacille Calmette Guerin (BCG), therefore the effect of irrigation could not be monitored in them. The remaining sixty-nine patients with first time low-grade superficial transitional cell tumors were studied for the effect of irrigation on tumor recurrence. There were fifty-three males and sixteen females. They were between the ages of 40-90 years old with a mean age of 62. They did not have any other known malignancy and were not treated for any previous diseases in the bladder. The diagnosis of the tumor was made at the outpatient clinic and all patients underwent a standard TUR with random bladder biopsies in order to exclude carcinoma in situ. In all cases previous to the operation urine cytology was sent and IVP was performed and was normal in all studied patients. Randomization was done after the completion of the surgical intervention by blindly selecting a note from an envelope which stated whether or not the patient should be irrigated. In the group randomized for irrigation, the irrigation was through a regular a 20F Folly catheter. In the group randomized for irrigation, instructions were given to irrigate the bladder at a rate two liters of distilled water every 4h for 24h.

5. Results

There were 69 patients in this study. Thirty-one were irrigated and 38 were not. The recurrence rate of the irrigated group within 24 months after the TUR was 8 patients 25%. while the recurrence rate of the non-irrigated patients during the same period of time was 22 patients 58%. The statistical difference between these two groups is p, = 0.0079 using a Chi square test .(The recurrence rate of the irrigated patients between 2-10 years with a mean follow-up of 6 years was 7 patients out of the 23 remaining patients 34%. While the recurrence rate of the non-irrigated patients at the same period of time with the same mean follow-up was 5 out of the 16 remaining patients 32%. There was no statistical significance difference between these two groups at this period of time. P=0.6119 using the same statistical analysis. The number of the primary tumors (1.2)was the same in both groups; so were the size of the tumors (1.7cm) and the mean age of the treated patients appearance of tumor which most probably occurs due to the continued insult by carcinogens to the bladder mucosa.

6. Conclusions

Water irrigation of the bladder following a TUR is very effective in preventing early recurrence of low grade papillary transitional cell tumors. It achieves this goal by mechanical expulsion of floating tumor cells and by preventing the cells from adhere.

Detection of tumors by Raman spectrum

There is a need to detect bladder cancer as early as possible in order to improve cure rateIn order to detect bladder cancer as early as possible to allow effective BCG treatment/ We conducted an experiment using a green laser to find the Raman signal os bladder cancer cells voided in the urine/ The use of Raman Spectroscopy in the diagnosis of bladder cancer from cells voided in the urine Urine cytology is expensive and inaccurate in detecting bladder tumors. The late diagnosis of invasive bladder cancer is a major medical and economical problem because bladder cancer is the fifth most frequent cancer in the western world. Today 85% of patients with high grade tumors, have invasive cancer at diagnosis. To address this problem we use Raman Molecular Imaging (RMI) to improve the accuracy of urine cytology. RMI is an innovative technology that combines the molecular chemical analysis capacity of Raman Spectroscopy with high definition digital image microscopic visualization. Digital imaging information and Raman Spectra show unique "Finger Print" Spectra of the different cells voided in the urine. The goal of this project is show that this method is accurate in the diagnosis of bladder cancer. Methods: Bladder cancer tissue with known diagnosis(10 Ta.G1) (10 T2-3. G3)and 2 normal bladders were scanned using a FALCON Raman imaging microscope. The typical Spectral Finger print of cells from samples of each pathology was characterized. Tissue samples were compared to voided cells in the urine and the same spectra were obtained from the same pathology. Further measurements on 45,49 and 50 urine samples from G3,G1 and G0 cases. Results: Using tissue, the G3 tumors gave a very high pick of scatter at 1584 cm-1 Raman shift. G1 tumors showed a less prominant but a significant elevation at this shift. While G0 did not show this elivation. Raman imaging showed that the material responsible for the signal was confined to the cells.

Fourty nine patients with no tumor showed 0% false positive results. In 45 patients with G3 tumors 44. (98%) showed the signal of a tumor and 41 (94%) showed that the tumor is of high grade. In 50 G1 tumors all were detected as tumor and there were only 2 samples that gave the high grade signal. In the RMI there is a distinctive difference between high grade and low grade tumors and non malignant cells. Conclusions: With this more reliable test it will be easier to find this tumor at its initial state. RMI shows that the signal from bladder cancer tissue and cells voided in the urine can be identified and distinguished from normal bladder tissue and cells in a very high accuracy rate and should be used in screening the high risk population.

This study was published in the January 2011 in Europian Uroiogy. This examination can be performed with the aid of a computer and does not require a pathologist or a Urologist. This presentation details the use of a software algorithm and Raman Spectroscopy to rapidly identify malignancy from cells in voided urine. The spectrum is analyzed by a software algorithm which removes interpreter bias from the analysis.

7. Methods

Cellular analysis was performed on urine collected from patients with and without TCC of the bladder. The urine was spun. The supernatant was discarded and the palette was suspended with distilled water. The process was repeated. The remaining material was placed into a Cytospin chamber which resulted in cells being deposited on an aluminum slide. Each slide was analyzed with the Falcon Microscope. The epithelial cells were photographed using 50x objective magnification. Raman spectra were obtained using 100 objective so as to minimize the empty space around the cell. At first spectra were obtained from 172 slides with an average of 5 cells per slide. The results led to formulation of the algorithm. Than the algorithm was tested on 196 additional cases. Results. The initial 172 samples were as follows: GO-50, G1-50, G3-50, CIS-22. Accuracy was as follows: G0-90%, G1-88%, G3-100%, CIS-95.5%. This analysis served to produce a software algorithm to identify characteristic signals produced by RMI. The algorithm was applied to another 196 samples made up of GO-76, G1-52, and G3-68 were analyzed. The algorithm's accuracy was: G0-90%, G1 57%, G3-97%. Conclusions. RMI of cells in voided urine can accurately distinguish benign from malignant pathology. Application of a software algorithm to the cellular spectrum rapidly and independent of operator bias segregregates benign from malignant cells.

Comparison of BCG types

Since BCG is the most effective treatment in preventing tumor recurrence we conducted a study to find out whether live bacteria or froze dried one is more effective Comparison of the efficacy and side effects of Pasteur vs. Connaught Bacille Calmette Guerin (BCG) treatment of Superficial bladder tumors One of the unclear area in treating superficial bladder tumors with Bacille Calmette Gguerin (BCG) is which preparation is the most effective one, and what are the relations between successful treatment and the side effects of it.

8. Material and methods

In order to find out which preparation of BCG 1) a freeze dried or 2) a fresh living suspension, are most effective and has a lower side effect Material and Methods: A controlled randomized study was done comparing the Connaught Imucyt to the original Pasteur strain. There were 66 patients in the study, 34 were in Pasteur strain and 32 in the Connaught strain. Each treatment consisted of 6 weekly installations of either 175 mg of Pasteur BCG or 108 mg of Imucyt. There were 50 males and 16 females. The mean age was 64 (39-86). Forty five patients had a papillary tumors, 22 grade 2, 20 grade 3, and 3 grade 4. Four patients had a stage A tumor and the rest had stage O tumors. Twenty two patients had Carcinoma In Situ. Results: In a mean follow-up period of 61.5 months the recurrence rate of The Connaught strain was 11 (34%) and in the Pasteur strain 10 (29%) there is no statistical difference between the preparations. The same amount of side effects occurred in both treatments. Not even one patient had to withdraw from the treatment.

9. Conclusions

Both Connaught and Pasteur BCG preparations are equally effective with the same amount of side effects. Sixty six patients with recurrent papillary transitional tumor or patients with biopsy proven carcinoma in situ (CIS) of the bladder were randomly treated with BCG following a TUR or biopsies for CIS. Thirty four were treated by a six weekly Pasteur fresh BCG (150 mg./ treatment) and 32 were treated with Connaught frozen-dried BCG (108 mg./treatment). Their mean age was 64 (39-86), 50 were men and 16 women. The tumor grades were: 22 grade 2, 20 grade 3, and 3 grade 4. Four patients had Ta tumors the rest had T1 tumors according to the ICCU calcification of bladder cancer. Twenty two patients had CIS. The age, grade, stage, sex were equally devided between the two groups. The mean follow-up time was 61.5 months (55-67) In order to find out which preparation of BCG 1) a freeze dried or 2) a fresh living suspension, are most effective and has a lower side effect.

10. Material and methods

A controlled randomized study was done comparing the Connaught Imucyt to the original Pasteur strain. There were 66 patients in the study, 34 were in Pasteur strain and 32 in the Connaught strain. Each treatment consisted of 6 weekly installations of either 175 mg of Pasteur BCG or 108 mg of Imucyt. There were 50 males and 16 females. The mean age was 64 (39-86). Forty five patients had a papillary tumors, 22 grade 2, 20 grade 3, and 3 grade 4. Four patients had a stage A tumor and the rest had stage O tumors. Twenty two patients had Carcinoma In Situ.

11. Results

In a mean follow-up period of 61.5 months the recurrence rate of The Connaught strain was 11 (34%) and in the Pasteur strain 10 (29%) there is no statistical difference between the preparations. The same amount of side effects occurred in both treatments. Not even one patient had to withdraw from the treatment.

12. Conclusions

Both Connaught and Pasteur BCG preparations are equally effective with the same amount of side effects.

13. Conclusions

It seems from our study that there is not any difference between the two preparations of Pasteur and Connaught BCG, not in the response to treatment, and not in the side effects. Therefore it is recommended to use any one of these preparations according to the convenience of the treating physician.

Lamm, DL., van der Meijden, PM., Morales, A., Brosman, S., Catalona, WJ., Herr HW., Solloway, MS., Steg,A. and Debruyne, FM.: Incidence and treatment of complications of bacillus Calmette-Guerin intravesical therapy in superficial bladder cancer. J. Urol. 147: 596-600. 1992.

Treatment of T1 Tumors

In high grade superficial tumors the recurrence of non BCG treated patients is about 90% in 2 years. With BCG treatment our results are: 40 patients with T1 intermediate (G2) and high grade (G3) bladder cancer were treated in Hadassah university hospital from 1983 to 2001. All the patients were treated by transe-urethral removal (TUR) of the tumor and additional Bacille Calmette Guerin (BCG) immunotherapy to the affected bladder. The mean follow-up to failure, death or to last examination was 120 months (12-228) . There were 32 patients that had no evidence of disease in this period of time. One patient was lost for follow-up 6 months after the diagnosis of his disease. 5 patients had invasive tumor recurrence and needed cystectomy 2 had recurrent low grade superficial tumors and were treated by a TUR. Four patients had metastatic disease on recurrence they all died within 2 years after the methastasis was discovered. They were treated by MVAC chemotherapy (3) or no treatment at all (1).

mRNA of IL2 and response to BCG treatment

We showed in the June 1996 issue of JCO that IL-2 is needed for the activity of BCG Novel Approach to Treatment of Bladder Cancer by Analysis of Interleukin-2 Gene Activation Carcinoma in situ is treated solely with BCG. However, 1/3 of these patients will fail treatment and suffer relapse. In lymphoid cells isolated from bladder cancer patients during BCG treatment, we studied the expression of two genes essential for regulation of an adequate immune response, encoding interleukin-2 (IL-2) and interferon-gamma. IL-2 and IFN-gamma are Th1 cytokines with many critical functions; they are essential for protective immunity and major players in the anti-tumor response. To this end, we developed a method that accurately measures the induced expression of IL-2 and IFN-gamma mRNA in peripheral blood mononuclear cells (PBMC) from only 10 ml of peripheral blood. Our finding is that the ability of the IL-2 gene to be activated is a highly accurate predictive parameter of cure from bladder cancer: 97% of patients whose IL-2 gene is inducible will enter remission. By contrast, up to 90% of patients whose IL-2 gene failed to respond to a stimulus had relapse or persistence of the tumor (Kaempfer et al., J Clin Oncol 14:1778-1786, 1996). Our findings strongly suggest that expression of the patient's own IL-2 gene is essential for mounting an anti-tumor response. This is the first instance of successful prediction of clinical outcome during cancer treatment, well before any symptoms of relapse. Determination of induction of IL-2 mRNA in a patient's PBMC provides feedback on the response of the patient even before termination of treatment. Patients showing a lack of inducibility of IL-2 mRNA thus can receive alternative treatment well before tumors recur. We propose to apply insight gained from analysis of IL-2 gene activation towards rescuing the 1/3 of bladder cancer patients that will fail standard treatment with BCG. Our strategy will be first to identify such patients by the inability of their IL-2 gene to respond to induction during treatment with BCG, and then to subject this subset to a second course of BCG treatment, either alone or in combination with human rIL-2. This combination of BCG and IL-2 was proven safe in a recent phase I study we performed and in a phase II study was more effective than conventional BCG treatment. Such an approach, we postulate, may elicit in these patients the needed anti-tumor response - at an early stage and well before relapse occurs - and lead to cure. We believe that our previous research creates an unusually strong basis for this project, which involves a close collaboration between a molecular biologist (RK) and a uro-oncologist (AS) at Hadassah Medical Center. From a scientific point of view, it will allow rigorous testing of the role of endogenous IL-2 gene activation in the anti-tumor response.

External IL2 and BCG treatment

As aresult of this study we tested the possibility of adding external IL-2 to the BCG treatment Phases I and II in the IL-2 BCG intravesical treatment of bladder tumors The standard treatment of superficial recurrent bladder tumor is intravesical instillation of BCG. The expression of il-2 is necessary for the success of the BCG immunotherapy. (Kaempfer & Shapiro JCO June 1966).

The treatment of bladder cancer with a combination of BCG and IL2

Using IL-2 along with an intravesical instillation of BCG has been shown to be successful when treating superficial bladder cancer along with BCG. We propose to find out whether the addition of IL-2 to BCG treatments will convert patients that would fail the traditional BCG treatment to responders of the combined treatment. A phase I study was undertaken to asses the toxicity of the Intravesical application of IL-2 to the bladder in concentrations ranging from 6 million units to 54 million units per treatment in conjunction with standard BCG (Tice or Connaught). Due to the considerable time involved with patient recruitment, phase II studies were done in conjunction with the phase I work. All 19 patients completed the Phase I study and all patients participated during the follow-up period. In the Phase I study, there were 20 repots of a fever higher than 38 degrees centigrade that lasted from 1-3 days in 10 patients. They did not need any medications for this side effect and it did not prevent them from completing the study (table 1). One Patient had severe arthralgia and fever 3 weeks after the last (6th) treatment and was treated with dual anti-tuberculosis medication and later by 3 Hydrocortisone injections. The response to the treatment was a complete recovery from the arthralgia. The blood tests for urea, electrolytes, liver and thyroid were all in the normal range during the treatment and follow-up periods. The cytology test for Bladder cancer was negative before, during and after treatment. Cystoscopy performed after the initial treatment at months: 3, 6, 9, 12, 16, 20, 24 and 30 were all free of tumors except for 3 patients. The recurrence happened in 1-3 years and all the patients did not quit smoking. The bladder was a bit red as observed following BCG treatment. 18

14. References

[1] Loening, S, et al: Factors influencing the recurrence rate of bladder cancer. J. Urol., 23:29. 1980.

[2] Deming C: The biological behavior or transitional cell papilloma of the bladder. J. Urol., 63:815. 1950.

[3] Soloway MS, Nissenkorn I, McCallum L: Urothelial susceptibility to tumor cell implantation: Comparison of cauterization with N- Methyl-N-Nitrosourea*. Urology, 21:159. 1983

[4] Wingo PA, Tong T, Bolden S: Cancer statistics, 1995. Ca Cancer J Clin. 45:8. 1995

[5] Boccon-Gibod, L., Boccon-Gibod, L., Desligneres, S., and Janin- Mercier .A: Bladder tumors: When to do and what to expect from random mucosal biopsies with reference to blood group cell surface antigens. Eur Urol, 13:1-6. 1987.

[6] Akaza, H., Crabtree, WN., Matheny, RB. and Soloway, MS: Chemoimmunotherapy of implatned murine ladder cancer. Urology 1983; 21:272-276.

[7] Shapiro, A., Kelley, DR., Oakley, DM., Catalona, WJ. and Ratliff, TL: Technical factors affecting the reproducibility of intravesical mouse bladder tumor implantation during therapy with Bacillus Calmette-Guerin.Cancer Res , 44:3051, 1984.

[8] Kirkels, WJ., Pelgrim, OE., Debruyne, FM., Vooijs, GP. and Herman CJ: Soft agar culture of human transitional cell carcinoma colonies from urine. AJCP, 78:690, 1982.

[9] Hinman, F., Jr: Recurrence of bladder bumors by surgical implantation. J Urol., 5:695, 1956.

[10] Kiefer, J.: Bladder tumor recurrence in the urethra: A warning. J Urol., 69:656. 1953.

[11] Moskovitz B, Levin DR: Intravesical irrigation with distilled water during and immediately after transurethral resection and later for superficial bladder cancer. Eur. Urol., 13:7, 1987.

[12] Pode, D., Alon, Y., Horowitz, AT., Vlodavsky, I. and Biran, S.: The mechanism of human bladder tumor implantation in an in vitro model. J Urol. 136:482, 1986.

[13] Pode, D., Horowitz, AT., Vlodavsky, I., Shapiro, A. and Biran, S.: Prevention of human bladder tumor cell implantation in an in vitro assay. J Urol., 137:777. 1987.

7

The Emerging Use of Smarthphone apps in Urology

Jonathan Makanjuola and Artaches Zakarian
King's College London, United Kingdom

1. Introduction

A smartphone is defined as a phone enabled for internet or email use. Mobile technology presents an opportunity for urologists to continue to lead in development in medical technology Urology continues to be a technology-driven specialty with the advent of robotic surgical systems this has led to urologists becoming the world leaders in the use of such technology [1]. Applications (apps) are downloaded items of software onto a smartphone which fulfil a specific function or role. The worldwide market for smartphone applications has grown enormously in recent years. Revenues from applications in the first half of 2010 were estimated at £1.4 billion ($2.2 billion), while in January 2012, Apple announced the twenty fifth billionth download from its App Store [2]. The Android market is the alternative to the Apple 'app store' developed by Google for Android OS devices [3]. Once downloaded, users can rate the app (out of 5 stars) on the app page so others can rate the usefulness of the app. Raters can also leave comment for prospective users to read.

2. Emerging use of smartphone apps in urology

Smartphones have the potential to improve diagnostic skills and education of a surgeon [4][5]. Urological apps available to download on the Apple App Store and Google Android Market are used for a wide variety of uses, including reference tools to aid diagnosis of urological conditions. Simple apps like 'Kidney 3D' a surgical anatomy tool and more sophisticated information apps like 'Prostate Cancer Calculator', a tool using a formula from Prostate Cancer Prevention trial to create a risk calculator designed to provide a preliminary assessment of risk of prostate cancer if a prostate biopsy is performed [6].

Urology apps have a broad range of uses like 'Advanced Urology' a urology reference app detaining the management of common urological conditions. There are many patient information apps like 'bladder pal' an app designed for patients to track fluid intake and urinary output. There are urological conference app like the 'SIU 2011 Berlin' app. It was created for attendees at the Société Internationale d'Urologie (SIU) conference where users can access the latest conference news, share contacts among the delegates; create a unique program for the conference based on the user's interests.

There were 69 apps found following a key word search of the term 'Urology', 'Kidney', 'Bladder' and 'Prostate' to the search tab in the Apple App Store and The Android Market. Included were all of the apps that are based on urological disease for health professionals and patients. Excluded were apps with a focus on Nephrology and complementary or alternative treatments in urology. The earliest posted app at the time of our search was on 19th November 2009. There was a more than doubling of the number of urological apps found on the app sites between 2010 and 2011. The average cost of the urological apps was £6.73/$10.64; (range £/$0- £34.99/$55.82), with 36 apps available for free. There were 52 apps produced by companies specialising in app development with 17 produced by Urologists. 35 apps were for reference, 18 for patient information, 6 for conference use, 3 for urology news and 2 for patient records in urological diseases. The types of applications are detailed in table 1. 65% of the apps found were aimed at physicians, 33% aimed at patients and 2% at urology nurses.

Type of app	Number
Reference	35
Patient Information	18
Conference	6
Urology News	3
Patient Records	2
Decision support	1
Drawing tool	1
Logbook	1
Social Network	1
Urology Careers	1

Table 1. The types of urological apps in the App Store and The Android Market.

There was an average 1 star rating of the entire urology apps reviewed. The app with the most ratings was Skyscape Medical Resources [7] with 696 raters and an average rating of 2.5 stars. There were a total of 8 comments posted about the urological apps (4 positive and 4 negative comments).

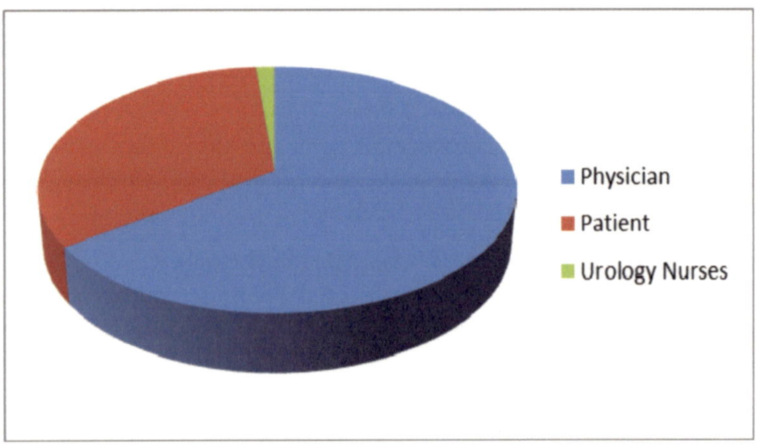

Fig. 1. The target user for urology apps in the App Store and The Android Market.

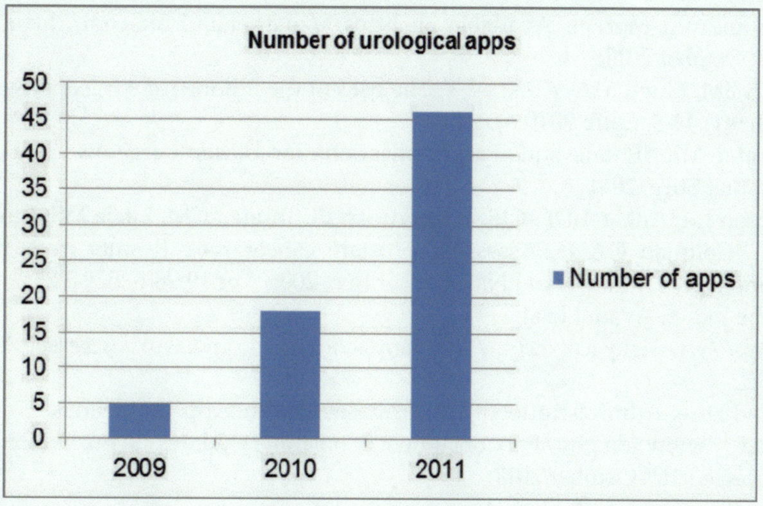

Fig. 2. The number of urology apps found in the App Store and The Android Market.

There is an exponential increase in the number of urology apps being produced each year. The use of these apps by urologists is difficult to determine by using the rating system provided by Apple and Android, as either they are not being downloaded or no rating is being left. As smartphones become an ever increasing part of modern life, healthcare is embracing this technological revolution. Urologists will be seeing patients who have read information on their urology apps, just like websites patients read before seeing their doctors in outpatient clinics. There are some negative aspects to the use of apps by patients and physicians. Regulation of these apps is lacking there is no regulation of the medical content. In July 2011, in an attempt to regulate medical apps the US Food and Drug Administration (FDA) are in public consultation regarding guidelines for the development a subset of mobile medical apps that may impact on the performance or functionality of currently regulated medical devices [8].

3. Conclusion

Apps provide an opportunity for urologists to engage with patients and offer a reference tool that can be accessed anywhere at any time on a smartphone. With this emerging market and increasing creation of medical apps, urologists in the future will be using more apps with focused urology content filtered to relevant and specific information. There will be an increase in patient information content in apps, presenting a unique challenge for urologists. This presents an opportunity for urological postgraduate bodies like the American Urological Association (AUA) or British Association of Urological Surgeons (BAUS) to lead the development of urological apps for use by physicians and patients.

4. References

[1] D Murphy, B Challacombe, M S Khan, and P Dasgupta. Robotic technology in urology. Postgrad Med J 2006;82:743–747

[2] Apple app store. Available at: www.apple.com. Accessed 02nd March 2012.

[3] Google android Market. Available at: https://market.android.com/?hl=en. Accessed 16th October 2011.

[4] Dala-Ali BM, Lloyd MA, Al-Abed Y. The uses of the iPhone for surgeons. Surgeon. 2011 Feb;9(1):44-8. Epub 2010 Aug 21.

[5] Freshwater MF. iPhone and iPad applications for plastic surgeons.. J Plast Reconstr Aesthet Surg. 2011

[6] Thompson IM, Ankerst DP, Chi C, Goodman PJ, Tangen CM, Lucia MS, Feng Z, Parnes HL, Coltman CA Jr. Assessing prostate cancer risk: Results from the Prostate Cancer Prevention Trial J Natl Cancer Inst. 2006 Apr 19;98(8):529-34.

[7] Skyscape Inc. ®. Available at: http://www.skyscape.com/company/companyhome.aspx. Accessed 16th October 2011.

[8] Food and Drug Administration. FDA Proposes Health 'App' Guidelines. http://www.fda.gov/ForConsumers/ConsumerUpdates/ucm263332.htm. Accessed 16th October 2011.